OTOLOGY MADE EASY

Essential Fives of Each Topic

UG/PG/DNB ENT/NEET

Dr. S. Mohamed Siddique

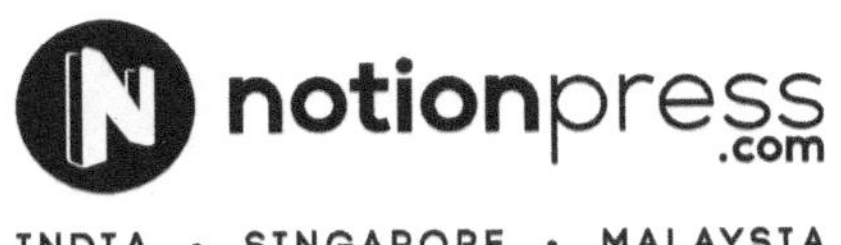

notionpress.com

INDIA · SINGAPORE · MALAYSIA

ISBN 979-8-89498-876-4

DEDICATION

Surah Al-Fatiha

(1) In the name of Allah, Most Gracious, Most Merciful.
(2) All praise is due to Allah, the Lord of the Worlds.
(3) the Most Compassionate, the Most Merciful.
(4) Master of the Day of Judgment.
(5) You Alone we worship, and you Alone we ask for help.
(6) Guide us to the straight path.
*(7) the path of those You have blessed; not of those who have
incurred Your wrath, nor of those who have gone astray*

This book is dedicated to my dear parents,
Haji T.S.K. Samsudeen and Amma Ponnu (Fathima),
my beloved wife Aiyeesha Banu,
my lovely daughters Reema Fathima and Reena Fathima,
as well as my cherished family,
Friends and teachers.

CONTENTS

PREFACE

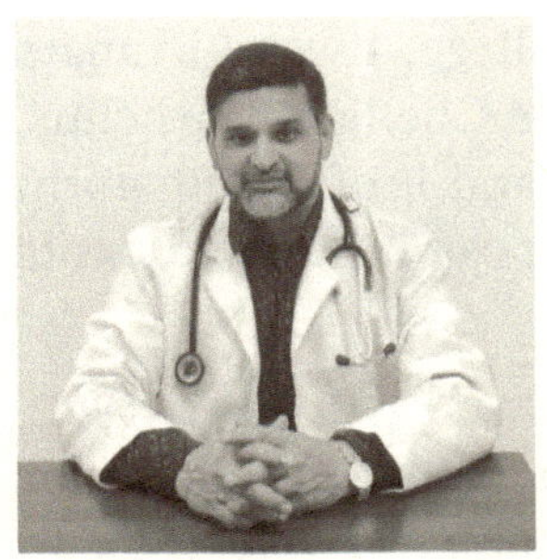

In 1999, I pursued a Diploma in Otorhinolaryngology (DLO) degree at Madurai Medical College, after completing my Bachelor of Medicine and Bachelor of Surgery (MBBS) degree at Al Ameen Medical College, Bijapur. Later, in 2004, I enrolled in the Master of Surgery (MS) program in Otorhinolaryngology at Madras Medical College. With almost 25 years of experience in the field, I realized the importance of sharing my knowledge with future medical students. This led me to the idea of creating a book on otology that would be a valuable resource for discussions during ward rounds, Viva, short notes in exams, and examinerled questions in practical exams.

I have a dream of publishing my notes as a book to help students and professionals in the field. Through this book, I aim to provide a comprehensive foundation in otology and equip readers with at least five important points for each disease and Definition of each disease in otology. These points can be used for ward rounds, discussions, vivas, multiple-choice questions (MCQs), short notes, and teaching. I hope to make the process of learning otology more accessible and enjoyable for everyone.

I would like to express my gratitude to God, my parents Haji. T.S.K. Samsudeen and Fathima and all the teachers and mentors who inspired me in my teaching journey. In particular, I want to thank Prof. Salim A. Dhundsai sir from Karnataka, who was my first teacher in medical science and made me repeat the points he taught in the classroom. I also want to acknowledge Prof Kannappan sir from Madurai, who guided me during my first Tonsil and Septum operation in 1999, and Prof AK Sukumaran sir, who helped me build my surgical confidence during my

MS course in 2004. I learned about mastoid operations from Professor N. Suresh Kumar, who is now the director of UIORL, and admired Professor G. Sundhar Krishan's expertise in endoscopic ear, sinus and Skull base surgeries. Later, as an assistant professor at Madras Medical College, I was fortunate to work with mentors like Prof Jacinth Chelliah Cornelius, Prof. M.K Rajasekar, Prof. G. Selvarajan, and Prof. M. Bharathi Mohan. I am also grateful to my MMC MS postgraduate students (2023-24), colleagues.

I owe a debt of gratitude to my inspiring 1990, 1991, 1992, and 1993 batch mates from Al Ameen Medical College for motivating me to pursue a career in teaching. I also want to express my appreciation to Dr. Janaki Raman for consistently enhancing our knowledge of ENT.

Dr. S. Mohamed Siddique, MS ENT DLO

Director and ENT Consultant & Head and neck Surgeon

Lakshmi Health center, Mogappair west,
Chennai, Tamil Nadu, India.

Associate professor, Senior civil surgeon,
Madras medical College, Chennai, Tamil Nadu, India.

E-mail: drsmdsms@gmail.com

YouTube: @drsmdsms

Phone: +91 9940254176

FOREWORD

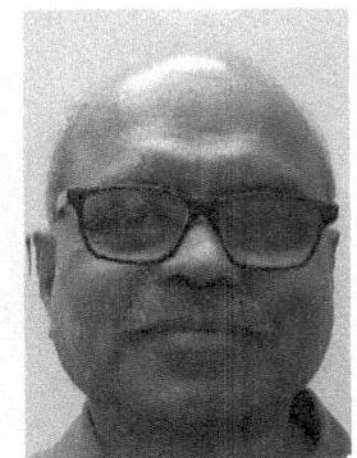

This booklet is an apt synopsis of otology that is extremely useful for students going for examination or viva voce! It is a quick revision to brush up and overcome the stress faced by the students. Dr. Siddique, being an associate ENT professor with abundant experience as an examiner and profound passion for otology, has strived to blend the mnemonics and rapid fire answers into a concised nutshell. I congratulate the author and encourage the students to make the best use of this book.

Prof. Dr. Jacinth Cornelius

Formerly Director &Professor of ENT, UIORL Madras medical College Chennai

FOREWORD

- It is both an honor and a privilege to write the foreword for this remarkable book authored by Dr. Siddique, a distinguished academician and an exceptional surgeon. Having been one of his mentors, I have had the pleasure of witnessing his intellectual growth 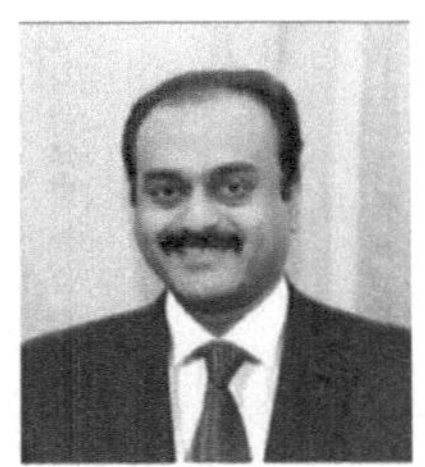 and professional achievements firsthand. Dr. Siddique's dedication to the field of otology and his relentless pursuit of excellence are evident in every page of this book.

- In the vast landscape of ENT subspecialty, the ear, with its intricate structures and delicate functions, stands as a testament to the marvels of human anatomy. "Must Know: 5 Key Points" is an illuminating guide through the labyrinthine complexities of the ear, offering both depth and clarity to its readers.

- The ear is not merely an organ of hearing but a sophisticated system encompassing balance, spatial orientation, and a gateway to the profound human experience of sound. This book meticulously dissects each element of the ear, from the externally visible pinna to the middle ear, inner ear and extends to the often overlooked, yet vital, blood and nerve supply. Each section is a journey through the anatomical and physiological nuances that underlie our auditory and vestibular systems.

- In creation of this comprehensive text, one must appreciate the dedication and expertise required to distill such complex information into a form that is both accessible and deeply informative. Dr. Siddique has succeeded in bridging the gap between intricate anatomical details and practical clinical knowledge, making this book an indispensable resource for students, practitioners, and anyone with a keen interest in otology. This holistic approach ensures that the reader gains a well-rounded understanding of the ear's anatomy and its implications for health and disease.

- "Otology made easy" is more than a mere reference; it is a reflection of the ongoing quest for knowledge and the relentless pursuit of excellence in the field of medicine. It is a reminder of the beauty of anatomical science and the importance of meticulous study in achieving clinical mastery. May this book inspire you to appreciate the complexity of the ear, encourage you to seek deeper understanding, and guide you in your medical or academic endeavors.

Prof. G. Sundhar Krishnan

M.B.B.S., M.S.[ENT], D.L.O.,

Ph D- Endoscopic Skull Base Surgery, Chennai

FOREWORD

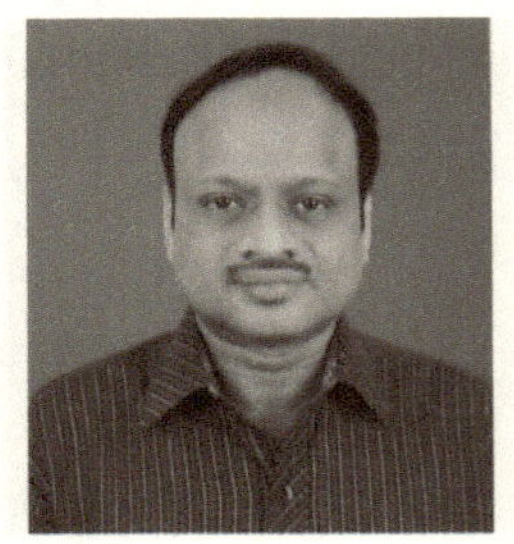

In the vast realm of medical science, few fields are as intricately fascinating and critically important as otology. The study of the ear, its functions, diseases, and treatments has seen remarkable advancements, transforming the quality of life for countless individuals. This book is a comprehensive exploration of otology, offering both foundational knowledge and cutting-edge developments in the field.

The human ear, with its delicate structures and complex functions, presents unique challenges and opportunities for medical professionals. From understanding the intricate anatomy and physiology to diagnosing and treating a wide array of auditory and balance disorders, otology requires a blend of precision, skill, and innovation.

This book aims to serve as an essential resource for both students and seasoned practitioners. It meticulously covers the fundamental aspects of otology while delving into advanced topics that reflect the latest research and clinical practices.

As you navigate through the pages, you will encounter detailed discussions on topics ranging from basic auditory mechanisms to sophisticated surgical techniques.

The dedication and expertise of Dr. Mohamed Siddique make this book a testament to the collaborative spirit of the otology community. His efforts not only advance our understanding of ear disorders but also inspire ongoing innovation and improvement in patient care. It is my hope that this book will not only educate and inform but also inspire and motivate its readers to pursue excellence in the field of otology.

To all the readers, whether you are embarking on your journey in otology or seeking to deepen your expertise, may this book serve as a valuable guide and a source of inspiration. Let it remind you of the profound impact your work can have on the lives of individuals, restoring not just hearing but also the joy and connection that comes with it.

Prof. M K Rajasekaran

HOD of ENT

Sri Balaji Medical College, Chennai TN

FOREWORD

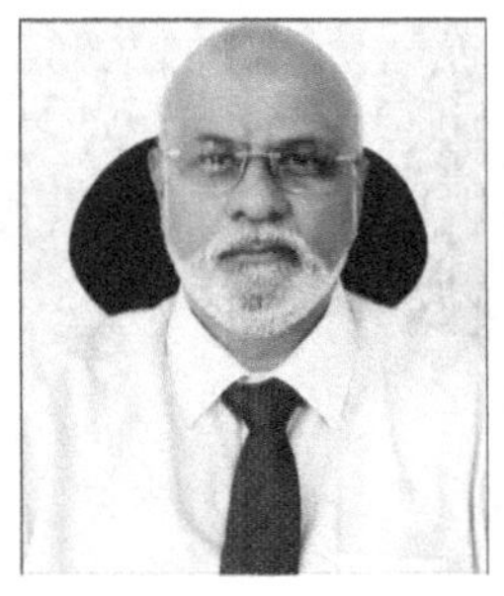

It is with great pleasure that I introduce this book "Otology made easy" written by Dr. Mohamed Siddique, tailored specifically for medical students for better understanding of the otological concepts in ENT. The author brings his experience to this comprehensive work.

In the constantly evolving field of medical science, the need for up-to -date resources tailored to the specific needs of medical graduates cannot be outstated. This book provides details of the intricacies in otology aimed to equip the younger generation to excel in this field.

From the fundamentals of anatomy /physiology to the latest advancements on the field of otology this book will serve as a companion to medical students.

I have had the privilege of witnessing the author's interest in teaching and his commitment to educate the younger generation. This venture is his genuine desire to show his expertise and inspire medical graduates.

I wish him great success and hope to see many more of his books in the future.

Professor Dr. N. Suresh Kumar MS DLO

Director, HOD of Upgraded Institute of Otorhinolaryngology

Madras Medical College

Rajiv Gandhi Government General Hospital

CONTRIBUTORS AND THEIR AFFILIATIONS AND ADDRESSES

1. Dr. Prof Balaji Swaminathan
Cuddalore Medical College Chidambaram, TN

2. Dr. Prof. G Selvarajan
HOD
SRM Chennai, TN

3. Prof. Dr. G Sankaranarayanan
HOD of ENT,
Sree Mookambika Institute of Medical Sciences, Kulasekharam

4. Dr. Saud Ahmed
Head of Department & Chief Consultant ENT
HBS Hospital
Bangalore

5. Prof M N Shankar
Rtd Professor of MMC, Chennai

6. Dr. Shaul Hameed G
Associate Professor of ENT
Government ENT Hospital
Osmania Medical College
Hyderabad, Telangana

7. Dr. Ahmad Abdul Khabeer

Associate Teacher

Gandhi medical College Hyderabad

8. Dr. Imtiaz Majid Qazi

ENT, H&N Surgeon

Rhinoplasty & Facial Aesthetic Surgeon

Kashmir

9. Dr. Sarafudeen PK,

Senior ENT Consultant,

Ascent group or ENT Hospitals, Kerala

10. Dr. Shakaeb Yasser Khan

MS, DNB (ENT)

BN Clinic 19

Kolkata

11. Dr. Nethra Dinakaran

Assistant Professor

Sri Venkateswara Medical College and Hospital, Chennai, TN

12. Dr. Prof. SOMU LAKSHMANAN

SRMC, Chennai, TN

13. Dr. T.D. Thimmappa

Government McGann Teaching District Hospital

SIMS SHIMOGA Karnataka

14. Dr. Prof. M Venugopal

HOD

ICH Egmore Chennai

15. Dr. Prof M Gowri Shankar

HOD

Stanley Medical College Chennai

16. Dr. J. Alaguvadivel

Professor

Department of ENT

Madurai Medical College. TN

17. Dr. Kiran Naik

HOD

ENT & Head and Neck Surgeon at Adichunchanagiri Inst of Medical Sciences and Research Center, KA

18. Dr. Jagannath B

Prof and HOD

Dept of ENT, KIMS Bangalore.

19. Dr. Archana

MBBS, DNB ENT

Chairman B.B. Hospital Chennai

20. Dr. S Rajendran
Professor of ENT and HOD
Govt Thiruvarur Medical College, Chennai

21. Dr. Nandini Devi Elangbam
MS ENT, Manipur

22. DR. Prof. Mohamed Anwar
MS DLO.
Trichy SRM Medical College Hospital and Research Centre,
TN

23. Dr. Praveen Kumar
Professor in ENT
Rajarajeshwari Medical College & Hospital, Bengaluru.

24. Dr. Vaishali Kataria
Mahatma Gandhi Medical College, Jaipur

25. Prof. Dr. Khalilullah. S
Head of Dept ENT
AIMSR (Apollo Medical College)
Chittoor
Andhra pradesh

26. Dr. Kannappan Alagappan
Madurai, TN

27. Dr. Rashmika Rajendran,

Assistant Professor,

Bharath Medical College and Hospital, Chennai TN

28. Dr. Gayathri. H

Professor,

Department of ENT,

ACS Medical College and Hospital

Chennai, TN.

29. Dr. Veerasigamani Narendrakumar MMC, TN

30. Dr. Vivek Mariappan MMC, TN

31. Dr. Saravana Selvan MMC, TN

32. Dr. Vinod felix Kerala

33. Dr. V. J. Vikram MMC, TN

34. Dr. Venkatesan Adyar cancer institute, TN

35.Dr. Ashfak Ahmad R Kakeri

Professor

Al Ameen Medical College Bijapur

36. Dr. Ashwin V G

Chennai

37. Dr. Seemab Shaikh

HOD, Dept of ENT,

Inamdar Multispeciality Hospital,

Consultant ENT Surgeon and Sleep Surgeon,
KEM and Sahyadri Group of Hospitals, Pune.

38. Dr. Vikashini MMC post graduate, TN

1

DEFINITION IN OTOLOGICAL TOPICS

EXTERNAL EAR

The external ear includes the auricle (or pinna) and the external auditory canal as it leads to the tympanic membrane. The auricle is an irregularly concave fibroelastic structure covered by skin that conducts sound waves to the external ear canal.

MIDDLE EAR

The middle ear is a non-collapsible gas packet contained within temporal bone extending from tympanic membrane, laterally and Cochlear Promontory medially, the middle ear communicates with nasopharynx antero- medially via eustachian tube and with mastoid air cell system through mastoid antrum.

INNER EAR

Inner ear is an osseous structure within the concise temporal bone that houses, both auditory and vestibular sensory mechanisms.

MIDDLE EAR CLEFT

It consists of the Tympanic cavity [tympanum), the eustachian tube and the mastoid air cell system, including the extension of the air cell system into the anterior and posterior petrous Apex.

TYMPANIC CAVITY

It is an irregular, air-filled space within the temporal bone and contains the auditory ossicles and their attached muscles

MASTOID ANTRUM.

It is an air-filled sinus within the petrous part of the temporal bone.

ADITUS

It is a large irregular opening leading from the posterior epitympanum into the air-filled spaces of the mastoid antrum, also known as aditus ad antrum.

ATTIC

It is an epitympanic cavity closed by partly bone(scutum) and Tympanic membrane (Sharpenell).

SCUTUM

Lower (squamous) bony portion of lateral epitympanic wall or outer attic wall

Also known as the shield of Leidy.

TEGMEN TYMPANI

It is the bony roof of tympanic cavity and it separates from the Dura of middle cranial fossa. It is formed by a petrous and squamous part of the Temporal bone.

PROMONTORY

It is a round elevation occupying most of the central portion of medial wall of middle ear and it covers a part of the basal coil of cochlea.

OVAL WINDOW

It is the fenestra vestibule, a nearly kidney shaped opening connecting the tympanic cavity with vestibule. The opening is closed by the foot of stapes nd it is surrounded by annular ligament Size- 3.25 mm in length and 1.75 mm wide.

ROUND WINDOW

It is a fenestra cochlea, closed by a secondary tympanic membrane that lies below and little behind the fenestra vestibule.

PROCESSUS COCHLEARIFORMIS

It is a curved projection of the bone (concave anteriorly) which houses the tendon of tensor tympani muscle and turns lateral to the handle of the malleus.

SOLID ANGLE

The angle between the 3 semicircular canal

FOSSA INCUDIS

It is a small depression which houses the short process of the incus and the ligament connecting the short process.

PYRAMID

It is a small hollow conical projection with its Apex pointing anteriorly. It gives origin of the stapedius muscle to the neck of stapes.

FACIAL RECESS

It is a recess bounded

Medially by the facial nerve.

Laterally by the tympanic annulus and Chorda tympani nerve

SINUS TYMPANI

It is the space present in the posterior mesotympanum.

Laterally bounded by facial nerves.

Medially bounded by the ampulla of posterior semicircular canal

Extending from Ponticulus to Subiculum

PONTICULUS

A) It is a spicule of bone that leaves the promontory above the subiculum and runs to the pyramid on the posterior wall of the cavity.

B) It is the central structure in the retro tympanum, it is a Boney ridge extending from the pyramidal process to the promontory.

SUBICULUM

A) It is a spicule of the bone behind the round Window from which it is separated by the posterior extension of promontory.

B) It is a smooth Bony projection that is situated posterior to the promontory and extends inferiorly from the posterior lip of the RW niche towards the styloid eminence.

PYRAMIDAL EMINENCE

It is situated at the center of the posterior wall immediately behind OW, It is about 2 mm height, Its base is fused with a canal of facial nerve. It lodges the body of the stapedial muscle and Apex gives passage to the stapedial tendon. It contains the stapedial branch of the facial nerve.

CHORDAL EMINENCE

It's situated lateral to the pyramidal eminence and 1 mm medial to the Tympanic membrane. This shows a foramen the iter chordae posterius.

STYLOID EMINENCE

It is recognized as a smoothed elevation at the inferior part of the posterior wall. It represents the base of the styloid process.

FUNICULUS

A ridge of the bone connects the basal helix of the cochlea to the jugular wall of tympanum in relation to the anterior pillar of the round window niche, that is, sustentaculum promontory.

FUSTIS-AREA CONCAMERATA

A small bony column mainly forming the floor of the round window niche from the promontory.

POSTERIOR TYMPANIC SINUS

It is a space present in the superior retro tympanum above the Ponticulus and medial to pyramidal eminence and facial nerve.

SUB PYRAMIDAL SPACE

It is a space present in the superior retro tympanum bounded laterally by the pyramidal eminence, medially by tympanum, inferiorly by Ponticulus & posterior laterally by facial nerve.

SINUS SUB TYMPANICUS

It is a space present in the inferior retro tympanum bounded posterior superiorly by subiculum, inferior and anteriorly by funiculus, posterior laterally by styloid eminence and facial nerve, posterior medially by Otic capsule and opens anteromedially to the round window niche.

BAST CREST

There are prominent structures on the medial wall of middle ear visible prominently during endoscopic ear surgery, this crest is a vertical bony projection (some people more prominent others less faint) extending vertically from cochleariform process to downwards.

ANTERIOR BUTTRESS

It is that part of the bone where the anterior bony canal wall meets the tegmen.

POSTERIOR BUTTRESS

It is where the posterior canal wall meets the floor of the external auditory canal lateral to the facial nerve.

FACIAL RIDGE

It is that part of the posterior bony canal wall which is lateral to the vertical part of the facial nerve.

BRIDGE

It is that portion of the posterosuperior canal wall which is lateral to aditus and overlies the ossicles and bridges across the notch of Rivinus.

NOTCH OF RIVINUS

The tympanic notch is a small defect in the posterior edge of the bony tympanic ring. This defect is located just superior to the tympano-mastoid suture line in the posterior ear canal

FACIAL RECESS

It is a collection of air cells in the posterior wall of middle ear laterally limited by Chorda tympani nerve and the posterosuperior quadrant of the annulus, medially the external genus of the upper descending part of the facial nerve.

It is also known as Chorda facial angle

INCUS BRIDGE

That part of the posterior canal wall, lateral to the fossa incudis.

COG

It is a bony septum that detaches from the tegmen tympani cranially heading vertically towards the cochleariform process in front of the head of the malleus, It transverse the ridge between anterior and posterior epitympanum.

TRAUTMAN'S TRIANGLE

The space bounded

superiorly by superior petrosal sinus

anteriorly by the bony labyrinth,

posteriorly by the sigmoid sinus.

CITELLI'S/SINODURAL ANGLE

It is the angle between middle cranial fossa dura and sigmoid sinus.

SOLID TRIANGLE

It is an area where the three semicircular canal meet.

DONALDSON'S LINE

It is an imaginary line drawn parallel to the lateral semicircular canal that bisects the posterior semicircular canal. Endolymphatic sac lies inferior to this line

SOUND

It is a form of energy produced by vibrating object

FREQUENCY

It is number of cycles per second

PITCH

It is a subjective sensation produced by frequency of sound

LOUDNESS

It is subjective sensation produced by intensity

INTENSITY

It is strength of sound which determines its loudness

PURE TONE

A single frequency sound

COMPLEX SOUND

Sound with more than one frequency

DECIBEL

1/10 th of log represents, a logarithmic ratio between two sounds, namely, sound being described and a reference sound, it is the unit of hearing

OVERTONES

A simple multiplies of fundamental frequency

WHISPER

The sound has to be heard at six meters

CONVERSATION

The sound heard within 20 meters

PINK NOISE

Number of frequency or less

WHITE NOISE

Wider range of frequency

MASKING

It is defined as procedure where the measure the quality of noise is delivered to non-test ear to prevent the artification of non-test ear

RECRUITMENT

It is abnormal growth of sound for example, when 40 dB sound is applied to diseased ear patients appreciate sound as 60 dB in Cochlear pathology.

TONE DECAY

It is reduction in responses of auditory system to sustain a continuous stimuli

Example: normal ear can hear continuously with the presented tone above the threshold for one minute and if it is neural pathology the patient cannot hear for one minute.

IMPEDANCE

It is resistance in flow of energy

COMPLIANCE

Opposite of impedance

IMPEDANCE AUDIOMETER

It is an Audiological investigation where resistance offered by middle ear structures to pressure changes in the external auditory canal is measured.

PURE TONE AUDIOGRAM

It is an electronic instrument designed for the art of ascertaining the hearing acuity (hearing threshold level) of a subject for pure tone sounds of various frequencies when plotted graphically is called pure tone audiogram.

OTOACOUSTIC EMISSION

Otoacoustic emission are sounds recorded in ear canal that are generated as a result of electro-motility of outer hair cells. They are used as objective tests to assess Cochlear function.

ELECTROCOCHLEOGRAPHY

The electrical activity generated by the cochlea and in the auditory nerve can be measured by a system called Electrocochleography.

BRAIN STEM EVOKED RESPONSE AUDIOMETRY

It is this recording of electrical activity of first ten milliseconds which is referred to as wave I to wave V, each of these waves, represent a neuro electrical activity generated by the neural generators at site in the auditory pathway in between the cochlea and the brain stem.

ELECTRONYSTAGMOGRAPHY

Eye movements can be recorded electrically and expressed graphically using a technique.

COCHLEAR IMPLANT

To replace a non-functional inner hair cells transducer system by converting mechanical sound energy to electrical signals that can be delivered to the Cochlear nerve in profoundly deaf hair cells.

BELL'S PALSY

Acute Peripheral facial nerve lower motor palsy that occurs due to viral inflammatory-immune mechanism. The disorder is self-limiting, non-progressive, not life-threatening, spontaneously remitting, and currently Neither preventable nor curable.

GLOMUS JUGULARE

It is a collection of ganglionic cells with thin temporal bone in close relation with the jugular bulb.

OTOTOXICITY

The tendency of certain therapeutic agents and other chemical substances to cause functional impairment and cellular degeneration of tissue of the inner ear and especially of the end organs and the neurons of Cochlear and vestibular division of the eighth cranial nerve.

MENIERE'S DISEASE

A disease of membranous inner ear, characterized by deafness, vertigo, aural fullness, usually tinnitus, which has its pathological correlation, hydrops distension of endolymphatic sac system.

VERTIGO

A subjective sensation of imbalance

NYSTAGMUS

It is a disturbance of ocular posture, characterized by more or less rhythmic oscillation of both the eyeball

DEAFNESS

Is a hearing impairment that is so severe that the child is impaired in processing linguistic information through hearing, with or without amplification.

OTOSCLEROSIS

It is a hereditary localized disease of bone derived from Otic capsule, characterized by alternating phases of bone resorption and formation. The mature Lamellar bone is removed by osteoclast and replaced by woven bone of greater thickness, cellularity and vascularity.

OTITIS EXTERNA

Any inflammatory condition of skin of the external auditory meatus

ASOM

Acute suppuration of Muco- periosteal lining of middle ear cleft

CSOM

Chronic suppuration of muco- periosteal lining of middle ear cleft

OME (OTITIS MEDIA EFFUSION)

A chronic condition where that is an accumulation of non-Purulent fluid within middle ear cleft

AURAL POLYP

Simple smooth edematous hypertrophy of mucosa of middle ear cleft.

CHOLESTEATOMA (PATHOLOGICAL)

A cystic bags like structure lined by keratinizing squamous epithelium containing keratin debris of variable thickness lying over fibrous stroma that has boney eroding capacity.

CHOLESTEATOMAS (CLINICAL)

It is the end stage of squamous epithelial retraction of the pars tensa or flaccida that are not self-cleansing, retain epithelial debris and often elicit a secondary, inflammatory mucosal reaction.

TINNITUS

The conscious experience of a sound that originates in an involuntary manner in the head of its own without external stimuli

PARACUSIS WILLISII

Patients present with conductive hearing loss appear to hear better in noisy environments usually because the speaker raises the intensity of voice and the masking effect of background. Noise is reduced because of hearing loss, seen in otosclerosis.

DIPLACUSIS

It is the apparent difference in the pitch of tone between two ears

Example: Endolymphatic hydrops

AUTOPHONY

It is an abnormal perception of one's own breath and voice seen in a patulous eustachian tube.

OSCILLOPSIA- perception that visual scenes or moving, usually during active head, movement and locomotion

EQUILIBRIUM

It is defined as the capacity of the body to maintain posture and spatial orientation at rest and during movement.

VESTIBULAR EVOKED MYOGENIC POTENTIAL (VEMP)

It is a relatively new vestibular testing technique that determines vestibular function by applying a repetitive sound stimulus to one ear and then averaging the reaction of the muscle activity in response to each sound click or pulse.

THE VIDEO HEAD IMPULSE TEST [VHIT]

It is an objective test of the Vestibulo-ocular reflex (VOR). The vHIT outcome parameter receiving most attention to-date has been vHIT gain, the ratio of eye movement to head movement.

MEATOPLASTY

An operation performed to widen the cartilaginous and or bony external auditory meatus. Names are

Korner

Farrier

Portman's

Fischer

Etc.

MYRINGOPLASTY

An operation to repair or reconstruct the defective tympanic membrane without middle ear work

TYMPANOPLASTY

An operation performed to eradicate the disease from the middle ear and to reconstruct the hearing mechanism without mastoid surgery with or without tympanic membrane grafting

OSSICULOPLASTY

An operation performed to repair or reconstruct the ossicular chain

CORTICAL MASTOIDECTOMY

An operation performed to remove the disease from the mastoid antrum and removing the block in the aditus and complete exenteration of all accessible mastoid air cells with preservation of an intact posterior bony external auditory canal wall without disturbing the existing middle ear contents.

CAT

An operation performed to remove the disease from the middle ear and mastoid by way of

1. Mastoid

2. Posterior tympanotomy

3. Trans canal route Followed by reconstruction of middle ear transformation mechanism

TYMPANOMASTOIDECTOMY

An operation performed to eradicate the disease from the middle ear and the mastoid and to reconstruct the hearing mechanism with or without tympanic membrane grafting.

ATTICOTOMY

An operation performed to remove all or part of the outer wall, (scutum) and the adjacent deeper post meatal wall to expose the attic and epitympanum and when, necessary the aditus and antrum in order to gain access to these sites and their contents and or remove drainage limited to these sites.

RADICAL MASTOIDECTOMY

An operation performed to eradicate disease from the middle ear and mastoid in which the mastoid antrum and air cell system, aditus, attic and middle ear are converted into common cavity, which exteriorization to the external auditory canal during the course of disease removal, the tympanic membrane, malleus, incus removed, leaving stapes in situ with footplate alone or supra structure.

MRM

An operation performed to eradicate disease from the middle ear and mastoid in which the mastoid antrum, aditus, attic and middle ear are converted into a common cavity, which exteriorizes to the external auditory meatus by wide meatoplasty. The remnants of tympanic membrane and ossicles are retained.

2

ANATOMY OF EAR

PINNA

1. Helix, Antihelix, triangular fossa, Scaphoid fossa, Tragus, antitragus, Concha and Cymba conchae.

2. The anterior superior portion of the concha is usually covered by the descending limb of the anterior superior portion of the helix. It is the lateral relation to the supra meatal triangle of the Temporal one.

3. Eminentia conchae-The medial surface of the auricle has elevation

4. It has 3 extrinsic muscles, 6 intrinsic muscles and 2 ligaments.

5. The Skin of the pinna is thin, closely adherent to the perichondrium on the lateral surface and thin layer of subdermal adipose tissue on the medial surface of the auricle.

"Darwin's tubercle-at helix Posterior superior aspect a Small tubercle"

DESCRIPTION OF NORMAL AURICLE

1. Average length of the pinna is 63.5 mm (males) and 59 mm (females)

2. The normal protrusion of an ear in about 30°

3. The distance Between ear and skull is 1.5 to 2 cm

4. Normal angle between concha and scapha is 90°

5. The average width of pinna in 35.3 mm in males &
32.5 mm in females

"Abnormal ear ->> 40 degree protrusion, > 2.5 cm distance, >
110 degree angle"

NERVE SUPPLY OF THE PINNA

1. Greater Auricular nerve C2, C3- supply lower 2/3 of medial surface lower 1/3 of lateral surface of the pinna

2. Lesser occipital nerve C2, C3- Upper one third of medial surface of the pinna

3. Auriculotemporal nerve- Upper two third of the lateral surface of the pinna

4. Auricular branch of Vagus nerve -concha, antihelix and Eminetia concha

5. Facial nerve-root of concha.

BLOOD SUPPLY OF EXTERNAL & MIDDLE EAR [ECA+ICA]

1. Anterior branch from superficial temporal and maxillary artery [Deep auricular branch and anterior tympanic Branch]

2. Posterior branch from stylomastoid branch of Posterior Auricular artery

3. Superior branch from middle meningeal Artery

4. Inferior branch from ascending pharyngeal artery

5. A branch from occipital artery

EXTERNAL CANAL SURGICAL IMPORTANT

1. 24 mm length, more horizontal in infants

2. Outer cartilaginous (8 mm) inner bony (16 mm)

Boney part formed by tympanic (anterior, inferior, lower ½ posterior canal wall) squamous part of temporal bone (upper ½ posterior and superior canal wall), cartilage part is elastic

3. Ceruminous glands, modified sweat glands, hair are present in cartilaginous parts. The perichondrium in the ear canal adheres tightly, so any infection can cause significant pain.

4. The Bony canal skin is very thin, lacking rete pegs in the dermal layer, which is the reason for flap tear during surgery

5. Keratin are shed towards the surface opening of the EAC from the Tympanic membrane

EXTERNAL AUDITORY CANAL

1. It is 2.5[24 mm] cm in length, contains Cartilage [8 mm] in lateral 1/3 and bone [16 mm] in medial 2/3.

2. anterior canal wall is longer by 4 mm than the posterior wall because of obliquity of the tympanic membrane

3. The auricle must be gently drawn downwards backwards for the best view of Tympanic membrane in neonate and children but in adult Upward and backward.

4. The rate of migration of the epidermal layer is 0.05 mm/day.

5. The cartilaginous portion contain Hair and glands

   a. ceruminous - Modify apocrine sweat gland

   b. sebaceous   - sebum

THE EXTERNAL EAR CANAL PARTS

1. **Tympani ring**-the medial end of bony canal is marked by a groove

2. **Tympani sulcus**-inner concave of tympanic ring

3. **Tympanic isthmus**-5 mm from TM where a prominence of anterior canal wall reduces the diameter

4. **Foramen of Huschke**-developmental defect in the Antero- inferior aspect of Bony external auditory meatus

5. **Tympanic incisura**-Notch of incisura- tympanic ring is deficient superiorly in the external meatus

DEVELOPMENT OF HUMAN EAR

1. Inner ear, which is the first Organ of special senses to become fully formed in man.

2. Otic placode formed at 22 days of intrauterine life

3. By the 25th week, the organ of Corti & spiral ganglion is completed.

4. Malleus incus Formed from first branchial Arch, stapes supra structure from second arch and foot plate from ectoderm

5. External ear canal develops from upper portion of the First pharyngeal groove and middle ear from Tubo tympanic recess.

WAX

1. The mixture of the product of sebaceous and ceruminous glands

2. Dry wax is yellowish or gray and is dry and brittle

3. Wet wax is yellowish brown and is wet and sticky

4. Wax contains amino acids, fatty acids, lysosomes, immunoglobulins and bactericidal products.

5. Secretion is affected by adrenergic drugs, emotion, fever and mechanical manipulation.

TYMPANIC MEMBRANE

1. 9x11 mm size, 55 degree angle with floor of the meatus.

2. Pars Tensa has

   – outer epithelial layer (stratum corneum, granulosum, Spinosum and Basale)

   – middle fibrous layer (superficial radial while deeper are circular, parabolic in orientation) so radial incision better than curved incision for myringotomy because of the radial Incision separate rather than cuts through fibers of the middle layer of pars Tensa

   – inner layer is a mucosal consisting of low simple or cuboidal epithelium to pseudostratified epithelium with cilia.

3. Pars flaccida (Shrapnell's membrane - has outer & inner layer no middle layer does not have annulus and has a single layer of pavement epithelium, so any lesion will not heal properly

4. Cone of light- Due to its angulation (55°), the posterior part of Tympanic membrane is placed laterally while the Antero inferior part in place medially causing the light to pass through the canal and reflect from umbo of TM towards Anteroinferior quadrant.

5. To see the tympanic membrane, one needs to pull the pinna backwards upwards in adults and backwards downwards in children (Because of the curvature of EAC)

MUCOSA OF THE MIDDLE EAR CLEFT

- Pseudo stratified epithelium- near Eustachian tube.

- Cuboidal - near facial nerve

- Flattened and non-ciliated - in the antrum

- Mucous membrane forms mucosal folds in middle ear (Anterior malleolar, posterior malleolar, anterior pouch of von Troeltsch, posterior pouch of von Troeltsch, anterior tympanic isthmus, posterior tympanic isthmus, superior incudal space, Inferior incudal space, Prussak's space, obturator fold)

- Mucus is produced by goblet cells and are of the highest concentration near to the Eustachian tube.

PRUSSAK'S SPACE

1. Medially -   Neck of malleus
2. Laterally-   Sharpernell' membrane
3. Superiorly   -   Lateral malleolar fold
4. Inferiorly   -   Lateral process of malleus
5. Commonest Site for Cholesteatoma origin

OSSICLES

- Malleus (hand, neck, Anterior process, lateral process and the handle)- Tensor tympani muscle inserted into neck of malleus.

- Incus (body, short & long process, lenticular process).

  During surgery, short process is more prone to injury

  Long process easily gets necrosis by disease due to tenuous blood supply

- stapes (head, neck, anterior & posterior crura & footplate) is smallest bone in our body - stapedius muscle inserted in to the neck of stapes incudomalleolar joint –saddle joint

- Incudostapedial joint - Ball & socket joint (to & fro movement, rocky movement & in and out movement) Hence all movements are possible.

- Foot plate 3mmX1.4mmX0.4mm (length, width, thickness) attached with fenestra vestibuli (OW) by Annular ligament

TYMPANIC PLEXUS

1. It is formed by the tympanic branch of IX cranial nerve and Carotico tympanic nerve of sympathetic plexus around the internal carotid artery.

2. Provides branch to the Eustachian tube, antrum and tympanic cavity.

3. A plexus on the promontory, a branch joins the greater superficial petrosal nerve.

4. The complete nerve passes through the temporal bone to emerge lateral to GSPN on the floor of the middle cranial fossa, outside the dura, it then passes through the foramen ovale with the mandibular nerve & accessory meningeal artery to the otic ganglion.

5. The lesser superficial petrosal nerve, which contains all the parasympathetic fibers of IX. It receives parasympathetic fibers from VII by way of geniculate ganglion. Post ganglionic fibers from the Otic ganglion supply secretomotor fibers to the parotid gland by the way of the auriculotemporal nerve (center is inferior salivary nucleus).

STAPEDIAL ARTERY

1. Stapedial artery arises from the hyoid artery (2nd aortic arch) near the origin of the proximal internal carotid artery (3rd aortic arch).

2. It Enters the Antero inferior quadrant of the middle ear and courses over the promontory and primordial stapes to form the obturator Foramen then proceeds anteriorly to pierce the horizontal facial canal into cranial cavity

3. It divides into - Maxillomandibular (Lower branch) Exit via Foramen Spinosum -Supraorbital [upper branch) persist as Middle meningeal artery

4. The proximal trunk of the stapedial artery normally atrophies whereas the distal portion of the middle meningeal artery persists.

5. Persistent stapedial artery as 1.5 to 2 mm branch of the petrous part of ICA, as a result of this anomaly, middle meningeal artery arises from the stapedial artery and foramen of spinosum is absent.

TYMPANIC CAVITY

1. Epitympanic cavity -Attic - Head of malleus & Body of incus

2. Anterior mesotympanic cavity - ET & carotid

3. Middle mesotympanic cavity – Handle of malleus

4. Posterior mesotympanic cavity (Retro tympanum)- stapes, OW, Long process of incus, IS joint, RW, Ponticulus, Subiculum, Sinus tympani and Tympanic recess

5. Hypotympanic cavity - jugular & Air cell mountains ridge

CHORDA TYMPANI NERVE

- It is a branch from the vertical part of VII CN, just 6 mm above the stylomastoid foramen.

- It passes from posterior canaliculus and run medial to tympanic membrane passes between incus and malleus, exits via anterior canaliculus (Huguier canal or Civinini canal) which in present in the medial surface of petrotympanic fissure (Glasserian)

- It joins with lingual nerves.

- It carries taste sensation from Anterior 2/3 of tongue to Tractus solitarius

- During surgery, it is best to cut the chorda nerve rather than stretching it.

ATTIC (EPITYMPANUM)

1. Superior: Tegmen Tympani

2. Inferior :   Ant & post. Malleolar fold

3. Anterior: Glenoid fossa of Temporomandibular joint

4. Posterior   :   Aditus to Antrum

5. Lateral   :   Pars flaccida below and scutum above

5. Medial   :   VII CN & Semicircular canals

Contents of Attic – Head of malleus, body of incus, Air

MASTOID ANTRUM

1. Medially-   Posterior semicircular canal, endolymphatic sac, dura of posterior cranial fossa

2. Laterally-   MacEwen's triangle (2 mm at birth, 12-15 mm Boney thickness in adult)

3. Superiorly   -   Tegmen Mastoid

4. Inferiorly   -   Digastric ridge laterally and sigmoid sinus medially

5. Anteriorly   -   Aditus in upper part, VII canal in lower part

6. Posteriorly   -   Sigmoid sinus

MASTOID AIR CELL SYSTEM

1. 20% of people have a cellular or sclerotic Mastoid. That's why we take x-ray mastoid for both ears for one sided ear disease to compare both sides.

2. Air cells are lined with a flattened non-ciliated squamous epithelium

3. Cellularity of mastoid is due to various theories

a. Endodermal invasion theory (Bast & Anson)

b. mesodermal theory (Schwarbart)

c. Mastoid plate destruction theory-pulling of SCM

4. Acellularity of mastoid is due do various theories

a. **Albrecht- A**spiration of meconium

b. **Tumarkin- Tube** – ET tube block in URI

c. **Diamant and Dahlberg-Dense** bone

d. **Wittmack-women** infantile otitis media

e. **Thorburn- A**nterior and posterior Isthmus obstruction.

5. Periantral, perisinus cell, peri labyrinthine, petrosal cell, dural, sinodural, peritubal, retrofacial and tip cells

THE TEMPORAL BONE

1. Squamous - MacEwen's triangle

superiorly: the supra mastoid crest [Which is the posterior prolongation of upper Border of the root of zygoma]

Anterior-inferiorly: – posterior superior margin of the external meatus.

posteriorly: A tangential line from the posterior canal wall cutting the supra meatal crest.

2. Mastoid- mastoid process and tip

3. Petrous- **Korner's septum**- it is Remnant of the PetroSquamous suture line. The persistence of septum leads to a false Antrum during surgery

4. Styloid process- 3 muscles and 2 ligaments

5. Tympanic parts form anterior, inferior and lower ½ of posterior external canal wall.

TEMPORAL BONE PARTS

1. Squamous- 2 surface [external & internal) 2 Border (superior & Antero-inferior) 1 mandibular fossa 1 zygomatic process.

2. Petrous -Base, Apex, 3 surface (Anterior posterior inferior), 3 Borders (Anterior posterior superior)

3. Tympanic -2 surface [Anterior posterior), 3 Borders (Lateral upper Lower)

4. Mastoid -2 surface (external internal), 2 Border (superior posterior) 1 mastoid process.

5. Styloid- 3 muscles [styloglossus stylohyoid stylopharyngeus)

   - 2 ligaments [stylohyoid & Stylomandibular).

CANALICULUS IN TEMPORAL BONE

1. Anterior canaliculus - chorda Tympani exit

2. Posterior canaliculus -chorda leave from VII

3. Tympanic canaliculus -Jacobson's nerve (IX)

4. Mastoid canaliculus - Arnold nerve(X)

5. Cochlear canaliculus- Aqueduct of cochlea.

STRUCTURES SEEN IN ANTERIOR SURFACE OF PETROUS BONE

1. Trigeminal ganglion impression

2. Arcuate eminence by superior semicircular canal.

3. Tegmen Tympani

4. Hiatus for greater petrosal nerve

5. Hiatus for lesser petrosal nerves.

MUSCLE OF MASTOID BONE

1. origin of Auricularis posterior
2. Origin of occipital belly of Occipito-frontalis
3. Insertion of SCM
4. Insertion of splenius
5. Insertion of Longissimus

STRUCTURE SEEN IN EXTERNAL SURFACE OF TEMPORAL BONE

1. supramastoid crest
2. Suprameatal Triangle
3. Suprameatal spine- Henle
4. Origin of Temporalis muscle
5. Groove for middle temporal vessels.

SUTURE OR FISSURES OF TEMPORAL BONE

1. squamo- mastoid
2. petro-tympanic: It lodges anterior ligament of malleus & transmits anterior Tympanic branch of maxillary artery and chorda Tympani nerve.
3. squamo- Tympanic
4. petro- squamous
5. The Körner's septum (KS), persistent petro squamosal lamina, is a bony lamina (developmental remnant) that extends from the articular fossa to the mastoid apex, above the middle ear, and runs inferiorly and laterally to the facial nerve canal. False antrum.

SINUS RELATED TO TEMPORAL BONE

1. Superior petrosal sinus - lodges in superior border of petrous bone

2. Inferior petrosal sinus -lodges in posterior border of petrous bone

3. Superior bulb of IJV - lodges in the jugular fossa

4. Petro squamous sinus- squamous foramen

5. Sigmoid sinus - sigmoid sulcus of mastoid process.

BAST CREST SURGICAL IMPORTANCE

1. It gives primary support to the cochlear form process (CP). The thinnest medial wall of middle ear over cochlea is present at the area of Bast crest Here the wall is 1 to 2 mm thickness

2. It is a remnant of the stapedial artery (stapedial artery in 35 % of cases passes in front of stapes, generally disappears at 2nd month of gestation. Bast crest is remnant

3. It is an identification mark for LSPN and Jacobson nerve. LSPN passes order CP and facial nerve through a foramen present at the top of Bast crest

4. In unidentified oval window in otosclerosis the cochleostomy window is made 1.5 mm below the CP along the Bast crest over the Scala vestibuli and piston is placed (Ugo Fisch)

5. Bast crest is the point for end of 1st turn and starting of 2nd turn of cochlea. Rule of 1 is firmly applicable to Bast crest* from the base of Bast crest the anterior wall of vestibule is one mm). The Bast crest guides surgeon the attachment of vertical tensor fold Hence the perforation

of vertical tensor fold is made above this crest to provide ventilation to attic in functional endoscopic ear surgery

POSTERIOR CANAL WALL RIDGES

1. Chordal ridge of proctor

2. Pyramidal ridge

3. Styloid ridge

4. Ponticulus- complete and incomplete

5. Subiculum.

INTERNAL AUDITORY MEATUS (MEDIALLY-PORUS, CENTRE –PROPER CANAL, LATERALLY-FUNDUS)

1. ONE CM in length lined with pia-arachnoid passes into petrous bone. (Hence, subarachnoid space extends up to the fundus)

2. Valvassori criteria - more than 2 mm different in size of IAM seen in Acoustic tumor

3. Bill's bar - separates VII from superior vestibular nerve.

4. Transverse crest (crista falciformis) separates upper and lower part

5. Structures passing through IAM

ANTERO SUPERIORLY- VII CN AND NERVE OF WRISBERG

POSTERO SUPERIORLY-SUPERIOR VESTIBULAR NERVE

ANTERO INFERIORLY-cochlear nerve and Labyrinthine artery

POSTEROINFERIORLY-INFERIOR VESTIBULAR NERVE (singular foramen)

VESTIBULE

5 mm x 5 mm x 3 mm

1. Anteriorly   - Scala vestibuli

2. Posteriorly   - 5 Openings of SSC

3. Laterally   - Oval window

4. Medially   - spherical recess (saccule), Vestibular cleft, cochlear recess (Cochlear nerve). Elliptical recess (utricle) and vestibular aqueduct.

SEMICIRCULAR CANALS

1. 3 SCC – lateral, posterior & superior+ 2/3 circle, unequal length- crus commune

2. Crista Ampullaris - sensory epithelium present in Ampulla of SCC

3. Superior canal of one ear lies nearly parallel with posterior canal of the other ear

4. Lateral canal lies nearly in the same plane which slopes downward and backward an about 30 degree angle to the horizontal when the individual is standing.

5. Lateral SCC   - medial to antrum, VII CN anteromedially

   Superior SCC - Apex is close to floor of middle cranial fossa - Arcuate eminence

   Posterior SCC - Donaldson line, medial to sinus tympani

COCHLEA

1. 2 1/2 Turn, height of apex is 5 mm (lower frequency)- 9 mm HEIGHT of base promontory (higher frequency)

2. Central cone or modiolus - arises from the cochlear nerve

3. Membranous spiral lamina divides the scala vestibuli [SV] above and scala tympani [ST] below (cochlear implant inserted into Scala tympani via round window)

4. Helicotrema - communication between the perilymph Space of SV and ST

5. The cochlear duct (scala media) is 34 mm in length. Reissner's membrane divides the scala vestibuli from scala media.

OUTER HAIR CELLS

1. 13,000 Cells, cylindrical shape

2. Stereocilia arrangement- W-shape at base, V-shape in middle & linear above at apex

3. Hair cells are supported by pillar cells, Deiters cells and Hensen's cell

4. Shorter stereocilia have fine fibrillar extensions to join inner hair cells

5. OTO ACOUSTIC EMISSION from outer hair cells, most diseases like noise induced deafness, and ototoxicity affects OHC.

INNER HAIR CELLS

1. 3500 cells, flask shaped

2. Inner hair cells are separated from outer ones by the tunnel of Corti

3. Cochlear nerve fibers start from IHC

4. Stereocilia arranged parallel to the axis of the cochlear duct

5. The shortest row of stereocilia in innermost while the longest row in outermost

VESTIBULAR LABYRINTH

1. The saccule lies in the spherical recess

   a. It is globular in shape connected with the utricle by utriculo saccular duct at acute angle & continues as vestibular aqueduct.

   b. It contains Macula sensory epithelium which is oval thickening on the anterior wall.

2. The utricle is regularly oblong in shape. It contains macula sensory epithelium on the lateral wall which is comma shaped. it has five openings for semicircular ducts

3. Three SCC each have an ampulla at one end. it has crista ampullary sensory epithelium which is a saddle shaped ridge

4. The saccule connected anteriorly to the cochlea by ductus reuniens

5. Two macula of utricle & saccule -> Otolith organ.

   otoconial membrane = otoconia + gelatinous membrane

ENDOLYMPHATIC SAC

1. Proximal portion or isthmus is first part wider than duct and lies within the bony vestibular aqueduct and lined by low cuboidal epithelium

2. The intermediate or rugose portion is the second part which is lined by columnar epithelium

3. The distal part of the sac lies between the dura of the posterior fossa and petrous bone. it is lined by low cuboidal epithelium

4. The distal part is surgically accessible in case of Meniere's diseases

5. These cells have absorptive or secretory function

COCHLEAR NERVE

1. Each nerve contains 30000 myelinated fibers
2. Afferent to brainstem, have their cell bodies in the spiral ganglion, the efferent to spiral ganglion, their cell bodies located within the brainstem
3. 95% of spiral ganglion are large type I cells
4. the efferent innervation is most dense at base of the cochlea
5. the cell bodies are bipolar

VESTIBULAR NERVE

1. 19,000 to 20,000 afferent fibers
2. Superior and inferior vestibular nerve
3. vestibular ganglion (scarpa's) contains bipolar cell bodies which lies at lateral end of internal auditory meatus
4. The human vestibular ganglion is distinct from all other species in that the perikaryon is not myelinated, instead it is covered by satellite cells
5. Acoustic neuroma arises from inferior vestibular nerve which has singular nerve as branch

FACIAL NERVE FIBERS – 10,000 FIBERS, OUT OF WHICH 7000 ARE MYELINATED.

1. Facial nucleus in the pons which receive pyramidal ipsilateral fibers (forehead and eye) contralateral fibers [rest of the face) then turns around VI nucleus
2. Motor fibers supply to muscle of facial expressions-buccinator, stapedius, digastric and stylohyoid

3. sensory fibers - nervus intermedius of Wirsberg via geniculate ganglion which is a unipolar ganglion supply to Conchal skin, supra tonsillar recess and areas behind the ear

4. taste fibers from palate & ant 2/3 of tongue to tractus solitarius nucleus

5. secretomotor parasympathetic fibers from superior salivary nucleus supply to lacrimal gland, nasal glands, sub mandibular and sublingual gland

FACIAL NERVE PARTS 50-60 MM LENGTH

1. Intracranial (cp angle) 10 mm - Thinner than VIII CN

2. Internal auditory canal - 10 mm- Antero- superiorly

3. Labyrinthine segment - 4 mm - Narrowest part 0.68 mm diameter (bell's palsy injury site)

4. Tympanic segment - 11 mm - medial wall of epitympanum.

5. Mastoid segment - 13-18 mm facial ridge

6. Parotid segment (extracranial) - between superficial and deep parotid gland.

BRANCHES OF FACIAL NERVE

1. Greater superficial petrosal nerve from geniculate ganglion

2. Nerve to stapedius tendon

3. Chorda tympani

4. muscles branches - postauricular, digastric, stylohyoid branches

5. Parotid plexus - temporal, zygomatic, buccal, Mandibular, cervical

BLOOD SUPPLY OF FACIAL NERVE

1. Anterior inferior cerebellar artery

2. Superficial petrosal branch of middle meningeal artery

3. Stylomastoid branch of posterior auricular artery

4. stylomastoid artery

5. posterior auricular artery, occipital, superficial temporal and transverse facial artery

CEREBELLOPONTINE ANGLE (BETWEEN PONTOMEDULLARY JUNCTION & INTERNAL AUDITORY CANAL)

1. Laterally by - Medial portion of posterior surface of the petrous temporal bone

2. Medially by - The edge of pons

3. Posteriorly by - anterior surface of cerebellar flocculus part of the lateral medullary cistern

4. Superiorly by   -   Trigeminal nerve Edge of Tentorium

5. Inferior by   -   IX, X, XI Cranial nerve and XII Cranial nerve

Contains – AICA (Internal auditory & sub arcuate artery), VII CN & VIII CN & Superior petrosal sinus, lateral sinus with jugular vein

3

PHYSIOLOGY OF EAR

FUNCTIONS OF EXTERNAL EAR [20 TO 20000 HZ]

1. Sounds conduction by

   a) Collection and transmission of sound energy

   b) Protection of inner ear by middle ear muscle

2. Pinna is a sound collector, intercepts sound energy and deflects it into the canal

3. EAC – gives Protection against physical violence and entry of foreign material by its tortuous shape, vibrissae and wax (gain of 2 dB)

4. Tympanic membrane -It protects the round window while feeding the ossicular chair and oval window. The Area of maximum displacement is seen near lower margin than central part of TM

5. Malleus and incus - rocking on a linear axis which runs from anterior ligament of malleus to short process of incus ligament.

   Stapes – Annular ligament is longer at anterior end than those at posterior end, side to side rocking movement is seen in an axis running longitudinally through the length of the foot plate

TRANSFORMER MECHANISM OF MIDDLE EAR

1. The amplitude is reduced at the oval window compared to the amplitude at the Tympanic membrane, the force of vibration at Oval Window is increased in the same

proportion

2. The ossicular chain lever ratio is 1.3:1, the malleolar arm is longer than the incudal arm. The malleus and incus jointly act as a lever pivoting upon the axis of rotation

3. The areal ratio (14:1) of Tympanic membrane and Oval Window - It is the Hydraulic effect. The effective area of TM is 2/3 of anatomical area as it is fixed all around the periphery in the tympanic sulcus

4. Overall ratio for middle ear [hydraulic)

$$\frac{TM\,55\,Sq}{3.2\,Sq\,Foot\,plate} = IT$$

1.3:1 X 14:1 = 18.3

5. Impedance transformation (IT) ratio = $(18.3)^2$ = 33.6

   "The ratio of acoustic impedance of air and water is 388.0. The impedance matching in middle ear less than ideally required"

THEORIES OF HEARING

1. place (Helmholtz) theory- Each pitch has its own Separate place on basilar membrane

2. Telephone (Rutherford) theory – discrimination of pitch depends upon the rate of firing of VIII CN and frequency is analyzed by CNS

3. Wever's volley theory- High frequency by place theory & Low Frequency by telephone theory. HF at Base of cochlear and LF at Apex of cochlear

4. Traveling wave (Von Bekesy) theory - initially the amplitude of wave is more at Oval Window and as it goes further the magnitude decreases and dies

5. Schuknecht - Pattern of neuronal activity by time, num-

ber of fibers, frequency of single fiber and selectivity of fibers

BONE CONDUCTION THEORY

1. Translatory or inertial mechanism- Ossicular chain vibrates at low frequency

2. Compressional mechanism(distortional)- bony labyrinth vibrates at High Frequency

3. Inertia of mandible (osseotympanic) - EAC vibrates

LATERALIZATION OF WEBER

1. Ambient sound theory

   The background noise that fills your space all day long. In case of conductive deafness, ambient sound is not heard, so tuning fork sound is Heard better.

2. Theory of dispersion

   All the sound from the mastoid goes into the inner ear and the sound is Heard better.

DISORDERS OF MIDDLE EAR FUNCTION

1. Total loss middle ear mechanism - 40-60 dB loss

   – No TM, No ossicles

   Reason- Displacement of Basilar Membrane by Vascular contents of labyrinth

2. The Round window baffle effect - 25 dB loss

   – No attic TM, No malleus, no Incus

   – preferential sound conduction to Oval Window is maintained

3. The Columella effect - 30-40 dB loss

- No Malleus, no Incus

- Tympanic Membrane Adherent to the head of stapes

- Areal ratio is maintained 14:1

- Lever ratio is lost 1.3:1

4. Tympanic membrane perforation   - 20-30 dB loss

    - Small perforation - Normal hearing

    - Large perforation - decreased Areal ratio 14:1

    - Posterosuperior Marginal perforation - 40-60 dB loss

5. Stapes fixation -   40-50 dB loss

–   increased Stiffness & increased resistance at Oval Window

–   Carhart notch seen in Bone conduction dip at 2000 Hz

Due to the loss of the middle ear component close to the resonance point of the ossicular chain

5 dB loss at 500 Hz, 10 dB loss at 1000 Hz, 15 dB loss at 2000 Hz, 5 dB loss at 4000 Hz is seen, this is due to "loss of inertia of the ossicles"

FUNCTION OF COCHLEA

1. Transmission - the transference of acoustic energy from oval window to the hair cells

2. Transduction - The sound energy pattern is converted at the organ of Corti into action potentials in the auditory nerve

3. Endolymph is the sole source of oxygen supply for the organ of Corti which itself has no blood vessels

4. Electrical potentials formed in cochlea

    a. cochlear microphonic potential arise is vicinity of

the hair cells being stimulated

    b. Summation potentials with high intensity arise from inner hair cells

    c. Action potentials arise from neuronal signals in cochlear nerve

5. Resting electrical potentials (endolymphatic potential)

Scala media (+) 80 MV

Outer Hair cells (-) 70 MV

Inner hair cells (+) 45 MV

Scala vestibuli (+) 5 MV

saccule (5 mv), utricle (2 mv) Semicircular canals (3 mv)

PERILYMPH

1. Perilymph is formed as an infiltrate from the blood vessels of spiral ligament within the labyrinth or suggests formation in the scala vestibuli

2. It is absorbed in the scala tympani or the existence of the aqueduct of cochlea which joins the subarachnoid space and peri lymphatic spaces.

3. Perilymph is chemically similar to CSF and extracellular fluid (High Na and low K)

4. Perilymph is present in scala vestibuli and scala tympani

5. Flow of perilymph up the scala vestibuli, through the helicotrema, and down the scala tympani to the round window, which bulges outwards opposite phase to the foot plate.

ENDOLYMPH

1. It is secreted by the stria vascularis

2. It is reabsorbed by specialized epithelium in the stria vascularis and diffuses across the Reissner's membrane to endolymphatic duct & sac

3. It is like intracellular fluid ($\downarrow Na^+ \uparrow k^+$)

4. It is present in scala media. The Cortilymph is present in tunnel of Corti, it is the intraepithelial accumulation of intra cellular fluid

5. Circulation of endolymph is radial flow (rapid process) from Dark vestibular cells & planum semilunatum to local absorption. Circulation of Endolymph is longitudinal flow (slow process) from stria vascularis to ductus reuniens to vestibular aqueduct to Endolymphatic sac.

LOCALIZATION OF SOUND SOURCE (NORDLUND)

1. Interaural phase differences are useful clues only below 1400 Hz (Low frequency)

2. Intra aural intensity differences are the basis for sound location above 1400 Hz (High frequency)

3. Time difference for complex sounds and transients

4. Superior olivary complex nuclei is center for both the ear

5. A degree of accuracy of localization from 5 to 17 degrees

CENTRAL AUDITORY SYSTEM - (CNS LIMCA)

HF-high frequency   **LF-low frequency**

cochlear nerve & nuclei	Anteroventral	-LF
	posteroventral	-LF
	dorsal nuclei	-HF
superior olivary complex lateral lemniscus	Medial SOC	-LF
	Lateral SOC	-HF
Inferior colliculus	Superficial	-LF
	Deep	-HF
Medial geniculate body	Lateral	-LF
	Medial	-HF
The auditory cortex	Rostral	-LF
	Caudal	-HF

JEWETT WAVES OF BERA

1. JI   -Cochlear nerve
2. JII   -Cochlear nuclei
3. JIII   -Superior olivary complex
4. JIV   -Lateral Lemniscus
5. JV   -inferior colliculus

FUNCTION OF THE EUSTACHIAN TUBE

1. Protects from Nasopharyngeal sound pressure
2. Protects from nasopharyngeal secretions
3. Drainage of middle ear secretions in the nasopharynx
4. Equilibrate the air pressure in tympanic cavity

5. Tensor Veli palate muscle opens the ET lumen while swallowing and only muscle affects the dilation of ET.

FUNCTION OF MASTOID CELLS

1. Air reservoir for middle ear cavity

2. Insulating chambers protecting labyrinth

3. May provide resonance to sound

4. THE MASTOID CELLS SERVE AS A RESERVOIR FOR PUS, WHICH IS WHY IT IS IMPORTANT TO REMOVE ALL CELLS DURING SURGERY.

5. Sound conduction

ALLAM CLASSIFICATION OF PNEUMATIZED SPACES OF TEMPORAL BONE

1. Middle ear regions - Mesotympanic, Epitympanic, Hypotympanic, Protympanic & Posterior tympanic area

2. Mastoid region – Mastoid Antrum, tegmen, Sinodural, perisinus, facial & tip cells

3. Peri Labyrinthine region - supra labyrinthine and Infra Labyrinthine cells

4. Petrous apex region – peritubal & apical area

5. Accessory region -zygomatic, squamous, occipital & styloid area

TAKAHASHI PRINCIPLE OF MASTOID

1. Ventilation, Protection, Drainage, Atelectasis, Effusion & Infections, are common in mastoid and lung

2. Middle ear ventilated by transmucosal gas exchange

3. Middle ear pressure regulation by gas exchange

4. Clearance & protection of middle ear by Eustachian tube

5. Both transmucosal gas exchange and aeration in mastoid are preserved when Epitympanic mastoid mucosa preserved

PHYSIOLOGY OF VESTIBULAR ORIENTATION

1. The Angular Acceleration in three planes of motion a) Yaw (Horizontal) b) Pitch (flexion & Extension) c) roll (Lateral head tilt about a horizontal axis). The linear acceleration in all dimensions

2. The labyrinth is on the horizontal axis of the cranium.

   - Lateral Semicircular canal slopes downwards and backwards at 30° to the horizontal

   - superior (or) Anterior Semicircular canal is anterior & roof to utricle

   - posterior semicircular canal is posterior behind the utricle

3. The Ipsilateral posterior and contralateral superior canals are the same plane. The ipsilateral labyrinth inhibit contralateral labyrinth by stimulus type I neuron of ipsilateral and type II neuron of contralateral which inhibit contralateral type I neuron

4. Utricular macula placed Horizontally and saccular macula placed vertically on medial wall, in utricular macula, the kinocilia are oriented towards the striola, In Saccular, the kinocilia are oriented away from the striola

5. In cristae of Lateral Semicircular canal, the Kinocilia are oriented towards utricle, [Ampullopetal) in vertical semicircular canal, kinocilia are directed away from utricle (Ampullofugal)

"Hair cells are depolarized by displacement of Stereocilia toward kinocilium Hyperpolarized by away"

CENTRAL VESTIBULAR CONNECTIONS

1. Vestibular nuclei lie on the floor of the fourth ventricle. No primary vestibular afferents cross the midline

2. DR   Dorsal (Roller's)

   MS   medial (Schwalbe)

   LD   lateral (Dieter)

   SB   Superior (Bechterew)

   Nucleus are groups of cell bodies, The Second order vestibular neurons

3. Vestibular ocular reflexes (semicircular canal-Ocular reflexes), otolith– ocular reflexes, vestibulospinal reflexes

4. a. Dorsal (DR) afferent from macula, Efferent to cerebellum

   b. Medial (MS) Afferent from crista, utricle & Cerebellum Efferent to coordination of head Eye & Neck movement

   c. Lateral (LD) Afferent from cerebellum & Utricle macula, Efferent to vestibulospinal reflexes

   d. Superior (SB) Afferent from cristae & cerebellum Efferent to semicircular – Ocular reflexes

5. Utriculo Petal deviation of the cupula of the Right lateral semicircular canal happens with utriculo fugal movement of cupula of the left lateral Semicircular canal then result in increased firing rate of right ampullary nerve and decrease firing rate of Left ampullary nerve

SEMICIRCULAR OCULAR REFLEXES

(LIRIO-LPS; L rectus I rectus I oblique - Lateral SCC posterior SCC superior SCC)

Example; Lateral SCC stimulates contralateral LR and inhibits contralateral MR.

1. Lateral Semicircular canal causes excitation of contralateral lateral rectus & Ipsilateral medial rectus

2. Lateral Semicircular canal inhibition of Contralateral medial rectus & Ipsilateral Lateral rectus

3. Posterior Semicircular canal causes excitation of Contralateral inferior rectus and Ipsilateral superior oblique

4. Posterior Semicircular canal causes inhibition of Contralateral Superior rectus and Ipsilateral inferior oblique

5. Superior Semicircular canal causes Excitation of Contralateral Inferior oblique and Ipsilateral Superior rectus

6. Superior Semicircular canal causes Inhibition of Contralateral Superior oblique and Ipsilateral Inferior rectus

Cawthorne / Cooksey Head exercises (5 minute three times per day for 1 to 3 months)

1. Stage I - Eye Exercises – looking up, down, side & focus

2. Stage II   - Head exercises – forward, Backward side with and with &   without   eyes closed

3. Stage III   - Head & body movement while sittings – Shoulder shrugging

4. Stage IV   - Standing exercises - get, up, throw a ball from hand to hand   while standing

5. Stage V   - Moving about – walking, circling, walk up & down and games

"Tolerance mechanism and the more diligently and regularly they are performed, the sooner will vertigo disappear"

4

PATHOLOGY OF EAR

PATHOLOGY OF OTITIS EXTERNA

1. Acute stage - hyperemia and intracellular edema (spongiosis)
2. Vesicle formation due to increase in edema which contains serous fluid with inflammatory cell
3. Vesicles rupture and exudes onto the skin surface
4. Parakeratosis - loss of stratum granulosum and corneum and production of nucleated keratotic cells which scales off
5. Chronic fibrotic and indurated phase

PATHOLOGY OF COALESCENT MASTOIDITIS

1. Hyperemia & neovascularity leads to-
2. Mucosal edema that leads to Obstruction of aditus
3. collection of fluid in the mastoid region under tension and venous stasis
4. Local acidosis causes decalcification of wall of the air cells because of dissolution of calcium - Halisteresis
5. Coalescence of mastoid air cells- mastoid will be filled with bags of pus.

PATHOLOGY OF CSOM

1. Lymphocytic infiltration and increased Goblet cells

2. Hyperplasia, Metaplasia and Polyp formation

3. Hyaline degeneration

4. Tympanosclerosis

5. Cholesterol granuloma - Chicken fat granulation

TYMPANOSCLEROSIS

1. Acellular hyaline and calcified deposits accumulate with in the tympanic membrane and submucosal layer of middle ear as **sequelae** of otitis media

2. Plaque occurs in areas where the gland and cilia are scanty

3. Formed by dystrophic calcification with calcium phosphate precipitate by change in PH due to fibrinolysis and hyalinization

4. Formed by matrix vesicle calcification by supersaturation of extracellular matrix with calcium phosphate due to fibrocystic degeneration.

5. It can be

    – Closed or open variety

    – Soft creamy or pure white hard

    – sclerosing mucositis or osteoclastic muco periostitis.

HPE OF CHOLESTEATOMA

1. The matrix - Epithelial layers like skin but more in quantity

2. Perimatrix - subepithelial loose connective tissue with collagen fibers, Fibrocytes, lymphocytes, histiocytes, plasma cells and neutrophil.

3. Cystic content - Keratin lamellae.

4. Atrophy, Acanthosis basal cell hyperplasia.

5. Epithelial cones formation in to the perimatrix

PATHOLOGY OF MENIERE'S DISEASE

1. Fistula of the membranous labyrinth

2. Collapse of the membranous labyrinths

3. Vestibular fibrosis

4. Sensory & Neural Lesions.

5. Organ of Corti – Loss of Hair cells atrophy of supporting cell & distal atrophy of tectorial membrane

HPE OF GLOMUS TUMOR

1. Red-pink to brown tumor tissue

2. Uniform rests of Zellballen of polygonal chief cell surrounded with fibrous & elongated cell

3. Round Ovid and vesicular nuclei 0.5 mm cell

4. Abundant clear or glandular eosinophilic cytoplasm

5. Neural infiltration IHC -> S100, Chromogranin, Nonspecific enolase

PATHOLOGY OF VESTIBULAR SCHWANNOMA

1. Firm well encapsulated mass.

2. Nodular surface

3. Gray or yellow and purplish mass

4. Antoni A – palisading pattern with large nuclei

5. Antoni B – Reticular pattern without nuclei [Verocay bodies]

PATHOLOGY OF CONGENITAL DEAFNESS

1. Aplasia & Abiotrophy

2. Chromosomal Aberrations

3. Antenatal - TORCH toxoplasmosis, rubella, syphilis viral

4. Perinatal - Infection asphyxia, kernicterus, toxic, hormonal and metabolic

5. Postnatal - viral, bacteria, neoplasm, hormonal, Environmental, noise, aging and toxic

"William Wilde was first otologist to recognize that Heredity played a role in hearing loss in man"

HISTOPATHOLOGY OF OTOSCLEROSIS

1) Active stage   - Otospongiosis – presence of vascular spaces containing highly cellular fibrous tissues with monocyte, Osteocytes & osteoclasts – Schwartze sign or flamingo flush appearance of Tympanic membrane

2) The Blue mantles of Manasse

3) Perivascular spaces become filled with projections of remodeled bone and around blood vessels

4) Decrease in osteoblast (bone formation) and increase in osteoclasts (bone resorption).

5) Final stage - Otosclerosis – High Mineralized bone with a mosaic appearance. vascular spaces are narrowed. New bone formation & lamellar bone is thicker and more cellular

5

MICROBIOLOGY OF EAR

MICROBIOLOGY OF OTITIS EXTERNA

1. Staph. epidermidis, Diphtheroids
2. Pseudomonas- common in swimmers, DM, malignant OE
3. Staph. aureus [BOIL] coli, proteus
4. Anaerobes
5. Fungi - Aspergillus

MICROBIOLOGY OF SAFE TYPE OF OTITIS MEDIA

1. Streptococcus Pneumonia
2. Haemophilus Influenzae
3. Moraxella (branhamella) catarrhalis - from pharynx
4. Staphylococcus aureus, Streptococcus Pyogenes, pseudomonas aeruginosa & coagulase negative staphylococci.
5. Virus RSV (Respiratory Syncytial) Adenovirus and Rhinovirus

BACTERIOLOGY OF UNSAFE CSOM

1. Proteus
2. Pseudomonas Aeruginosa
3. Staphylococcus aureus

4.   Escherichia coli (Faecal - Oral route)

5.   Bacteroides melaninogenicus & fragilis

TUBERCULOSIS OTITIS MEDIA (5P'S)

1.   Painless otorrhea

2.   Pale exuberant granulation

3.   Multiple Perforation of Tympanic membrane

4.   Tympanic membrane looks rosy pink in Early stage and later yellowish white

5.   Facial Palsy, Post aural fistula or abscess & Hearing loss

6

RADIOLOGY OF EAR

X-MASTOID VIEWS

1. Law's view (oblique Lateral Stockholm B)
2. Submento vertical (Axial view)
3. Schuller's view (Lateral)
4. Stenver"s view (oblique posteroanterior)
5. Guillen's view (Transorbital)

IMPORTANCE OF X-RAY MASTOID

1. Anatomical variation - Low lying dura, forward lying sinus
2. To see for Bony erosions
3. Extent of Pneumatization
4. To see for cavity
5. Sclerosis/ clouding of mastoid

X-RAY FINDING IN CHOLESTEATOMA CAVITY

1. Smooth margins
2. Cotton wool appearance
3. Cavity seen in mastoid area
4. Mastoid sclerosis is present
5. Mild osteitis around the margin of cavity->hyperdense due to inflammation

X-RAY FINDING IN OPERATED CAVITY

1. Irregular margins due to osteogenesis
2. Homogeneous Appearance
3. Cavity seen mastoid and middle ear area
4. Sclerosis is absent
5. No Osteitis feature seen

DD OF MASTOID CAVITY (CAVIT SOME)

1. **Cholesteatoma, Cholesterol granuloma and chronic foreign body**
2. **Antrum(large) cell**
3. **Vascular - Glomus and High jugular bulb, facial neuroma**
4. **Iatrogenic-post-operative cavity**
5. **Tuberculosis, sarcoidosis**

   secondary deposit Metastasis, Multiple myeloma, and Eosinophilic granuloma

HRCT -TEMPORAL BONE

1. 1 or 2 mm sections high resolution mode on "Bone Algorithm"
2. These are viewed on a wide window setting of 3000-4000 HU
3. Axial section
   1) Lower section   - Base of cochlea, RW niche
   2) Higher section

      mid-modiolus, stapes, ow & vestibule
   3) 2nd part of VII nerve section – IAM

4) Lateral semicircular section – Crura of stapes & IAM

1. Coronal Section

    5) Level of carotid canal   - Cochlea, malleus

    6) Level of Vestibule   - IAM, Stapes & OW

    7) Level of SCC   - LSC, Pyramidal Eminence Facial recess & Sinus tympani

    8) Level of Mastoid   - Descending facial canal jugular fossa and Posterior semicircular canal

2. CT - Intravenous contrast indicated in Glomus tumor

    (50 ml of Iodine containing contrast medium)

"Contrast Enhancement is almost never used for lesions of the petrous temporal Bone"

CT- SCAN FINDING OF CHOLESTEATOMA

1. Scutum erosion is earliest sign

2. Soft tissue mass with homogeneous opacity

3. Normal figure pattern of eight is lost due to erosion of lateral wall of attic

4. Erosion of ossicles

5. Erosion of Facial canal & Labyrinth.

RADIOLOGICAL ASSESSMENT OF "RISING SUN BEHIND THE DRUM"

1. Axial CT - Jugular fossa enlarged with cortex eroded-Glomus jugulare

2. Axial CT - Jugular Fossa Enlarged without cortex eroded-High Jugular bulb

3. Axial CT - Jugular fossa is normal go for coronal CT

4. Coronal CT - Normal carotid canal-Glomus tympani

5. Coronal CT - Laterally placed carotid canal-Aberrant Carotid artery

RADIONUCLIDE SCAN

1. To differentiate between a suspected inflammatory lesion and a Neoplastic lesion.

2. Scan technique is to do an early (1 hours) and late (3 hours) scanning procedure

3. Inflammation, there will be ↑ uptake within 1 hrs in soft tissue and ↓ uptake after 3 hours

4. Neoplasm, there will be ↑ uptake in 1 hours and ↑↑ uptake after 3 hours also

5. Necrotizing otitis externa, there will be ↑ uptake in 1 hours same uptake after 3 hours also

7

TYMPANIC MEMBRANE FINDING IN OTOLOGICAL DISEASES

TM FINDINGS IN OTITIS MEDIA WITH EFFUSION

1) Loss of Translucency ranging from pale gray or amber to black or

   blue drum –increased vascularity

2) TM is thickened dull and opalescent or thin & reflective

3) Fluid levels or air bubbles are visible

4) Splitting and derangement of the light reflex with retraction of the pars tensa

5) Rotation and displacement of malleus handle with prominence of the lateral process of the malleus

TM FINDINGS IN RETRACTED TM

1) Dull and lusterless intact TM

2) Core of light distorted or absent

3) Apparent Shortening of handle of malleus

4) Prominent ossicles

5) Prominent malleolar folds

TM FINDINGS IN ATELECTATIC OTITIS MEDIA (STAGE LLL PARS TENSA RETRACTION)

1) Retracted intact TM

2) TM is thin and atrophic due to decreased fibrous component

3) Incus / malleus can be seen clearly when tympanic membrane is collapsed

4) Collapse of Wide - atrophic membrane over the lenticular process of incus, stapes & promontory

5) Tympanic membrane is not adherent to the medial wall of the Middle ear and the mucosal lining of the middle ear is intact.

FINDINGS IN ADHESIVE OTITIS MEDIA (STAGE LV PARS TENSA RETRACTION)

1) Dull, Lusterless intact Tympanic membrane

2) Absent cone of light

3) TM movement is absent on Seigel's pneumatic speculum

4) Long process of incus necrosis due to

1. Poor Blood Supply

2. Low grade osteitis by increased vascularity

5) Tympanic membrane is adherent to the medial wall of the Middle ear and the mucosal lining of the middle ear.

TYMPANIC MEMBRANE FINDINGS IN TYMPANOSCLEROSIS

1) Intact Mobile or immobile TM

2) Chalky white area seen on TM

3) cone of light is absent or present

4) Acellular hyaline and calcified deposits accumulate within the tympanic membrane and submucosa of middle ear

5) Can occur in Tympanic membrane/Oval Window/ Round window/Ossicles and fallopian tube.

TYMPANIC MEMBRANE FINDINGS IN ACUTE SUPPURATIVE OTITIS MEDIA

1) Stage of hyperemia - Tympanic membrane congested

2) Stage of Exudation - bulging of TM, cart wheel appearance

3) Stage of suppuration - Small perforation

4) Stage of coalescence - central perforation with sagging of the posterior superior metal wall due to periosteal thickening and subperiosteal abscess

5) Stage of complication and resolution - signs depend on the type of complication & resolution

TYMPANIC MEMBRANE FINDING IN CHRONIC SUPPURATIVE OTITIS MEDIA

1) Healed otitis media - Scarring, thickening normal TM

2) inactive (mucosal) com - Permanent defects of pars tensa without evidence of inflammation

3) Active (mucosal) com- TM perforation in pars tensa,

   Middle ear mucosa is Inflamed,

   granulation or polyps are seen and

   mucopurulent discharge present.

4) Active squamous com - Cholesteatoma seen with pars flaccida and pars tensa perforation

5) Inactive squamous com - Retraction pocket in pars flaccida and

   – Posterosuperior part of pars tensa

   – Fundus of pocket seen

- Debris seen but self-cleaning cavity

TYMPANIC MEMBRANE FINDING IN MIDDLE EAR BAROTRAUMA

1. Grade I - Redness and retraction of TYMPANIC MEMBRANE

2. Grade II - Slight Hemorrhage with in the TYMPANIC MEMBRANE

3. Grade III - Gross Hemorrhage with in the Tympanic membrane

4. Grade IV - Tympanic membrane bulge with free blood in middle ear

5. Grade V - Tympanic membrane perforation with Hemorrhage in middle ear.

TYMPANIC MEMBRANE FINDING IN OTOSCLEROSIS

1. Tympanic membrane is Normal to atrophic, Thickened, rigid or immobile

2. Flamingo flush or Schwartze sign as result of vascular bone on promontory [Active disease)

3. Cone of light is present

4. No fluid in the middle ear and 5. No discharge seen in the external canal.

TUBOTYMPANIC TYPE OF CSOM

1) Intermittent, mucopurulent discharge non foul smell, moderate to profuse amount discharge, non-blood-stained discharge

2) single central perforation (multiple perforation seen in TB) with Regular margin in pars tensa [irregular margin

seen in traumatic perforation]

3) Ear discharge aggravated by URI or when water enter to ear and relieved with medication

4) Active stage, Quiescent stage, inactive stage and healed stage

5) Through the perforation middle ear mucosa can be found to be congested or have polypoidal mucosa or granulation

TM FINDING IN SUBTOTAL PERFORATION

1) Tympanic annulus only seen

2) Foreshortening of malleus handle and is tethered to the promontory

3) Floor of middle ear in marked by mountainous ridges, spikes and valleys draped in mucosa (Mastoid air cell system)

4) Eustachian tube opening & Round window are seen

5) Ossicular chain may be absent example: long process of incus & middle ear mucosa congested or normal

"In total perforation, the tympanic annulus not seen"

ATTICO ANTRAL TYPE OF CSOM

1) Thick, purulent, scanty, foul smelling, bloodstained persistent discharge

2) The discharge is not aggravated by URI

3) Perforation seen in pars flaccida or Posterosuperior part of pars tensa

4) Cholesteatoma flakes

5) Granulation and attic scutum erosion seen with fishy odor & posterior marginal pathology like osteitis seen.

STAGING OF ATTIC RETRACTION – TOS CLASSIFICATION

1) Type O -> Normal pars flaccida

2) Type I -> Retraction not in contact with the malleus neck

3) Type II -> Pars flaccida contact with malleus neck

4) Type III -> Limited(partial) outer attic wall erosion (scutum)

5) Type IV -> Total outer attic wall erosion (scutum)

STAGING OF PARS TENSA RETRACTION - SADE CLASSIFICATION

1) Grade I - Normal tympanic membrane

2) Grade II - Retraction in contact with handle of malleus

3) Grade III - TM in contact with Medial wall of middle ear but mobility present

4) Grade IV - Tympanic membrane mobility absent

5) There will be temporary partial hearing loss in Eustachian catarrh

8

CASE PRESENTATION AND DISCUSSION

EAR DISCHARGE - OTORRHOEA

1. Watery — CSF, Trauma, Otomycosis and Otitis Externa
2. Serous — Allergic otitis externa, TB
3. Mucopurulent — CSOM (tubo tympanic)
4. Purulent — CSOM (ATTICO ANTRAL) Cholesteatoma
5. Blood stained — Malignancy, Granulation, Glomus

WHY IS ATTIC DISEASE DANGEROUS?

1. lined by single layer of pavement epithelium (cuboidal without basement membrane)
2. Minimum ventilation & improper Drainage
3. Crowded Structures- Head of malleolus and Body of incus
4. Lateral wall related to bone - scutum erosion
5. Middle cranial fossa, aditus are close to attic, so, disease spreads early and leads to intracranial complications

REASON FOR EAR DISCHARGE/ CHARACTERS

1. Profuse discharge due to more goblet cell
2. Scanty discharge due to epithelium shedding

3. Mucopurulent due to Gram positive bacteria

4. Purulent due to anaerobic infection

5. Foul smell and bloodstains discharge due to osteitis and secondary bacterial infection.

THREE FINGER TEST

1. Index, middle and thumb are used

2. Index finger is applied over mastoid process tip - tenderness indicates mastoiditis

3. Middle finger is applied over the concha - tenderness indicates inflammation in the mastoid antrum area

4. Thumb is used to apply pressure over the posterior aspect of mastoid Tenderness indicates mastoid emissary veins thrombophlebitis

5. Present in Acute mastoiditis.

CAUSES OF MASTOID CAVITY PROBLEM

1. Large mastoid cavity

2. Improper meatoplasty

3. High facial ridge and inadequate removal of Bridge

4. Lining of the respiratory mucus secreting epithelium

5. Recidivism- Residual or Recurrent Cholesteatoma

METHOD OF VISUALIZES THE FUNDUS OF RETRACTION POCKET

1. Probing with Right angled instrument

2. Toynbee maneuver

3. Valsalva maneuver

4. O to Endoscopic examination

6. springel boric powder.

DIFFERENTIAL DIAGNOSIS OF POLYPOID MASS OF EAC

1. Aural polyp

2. Osteoma & carcinoma

3. Papilloma & ceruminoma

4. Glomus & Rhinosporidiosis

5. Malignancy

FACTORS RESPONSIBLE FOR A SUCCESSFUL MYRINGOPLASTY

1. Aseptic technique

2. Eradication of the Focus of Infection

3. Functioning Eustachian tube

4. Well aerated middle ear cleft

5. preservation of tympanic annulus

RED TYMPANIC MEMBRANE

1. Trauma and barotrauma

2. Chronic serous otitis media

3. cholesterol granuloma and reparative granuloma

4. Glomus jugulare and aberrant carotid artery

5. Leukemia

WHITE TYMPANIC MEMBRANE

1. Tympanosclerosis

2. Adhesive otitis media

3. Atelectatic Tympanic membrane or thinned tympanic membrane

4. Scar in the Tympanic membrane

5. Congenital cholesteatoma

REASON FOR SAFE TYPE OF (TUBO TYMPANIC) CSOM

1. Less migration of squamous epithelium due to intact remaining Tympanic membrane

2. No important Structure present in anterior inferior quadrant of Tympanic membrane

3. Frequent clearing of infection by ciliary action

4. Mucosal lining is thick pseudostratified ciliated columnar epithelium

5. Complications of disease is rare

AURAL POLYP - PALE IN COLOR

1. Hyperplasia edematous mucosa of middle ear cleft

2. Arise from any part of middle Ear cleft

3. Covered by stratified squamous Epithelium

4. Insensitive to touch and mobile

5. Does not bleed on touch associated with safe type (tubo tympanic) CSOM.

AURAL GRANULATION - RED IN COLOR

1. Hyperemic mucosa with osteitis (Cholesteatoma underlying it)

2. Arise from non-draining areas of middle Ear cleft

3. Not covered by epithelium and covered by fibroblasts with budding epithelium

4. Sensitive to touch & not mobile

5. Bleeds on touch associated with unsafe (attico antral) type of CSOM

REASON FOR GROWTH OF SQUAMOUS EPITHELIUM IN PERFORATION

1. Persistent discharge

2. Endothelium cannot survive in External environment towards the external auditory canal

3. Squamous Epithelium grows faster

4. Endothelium cells damaged due to repeated infection

5. Contact inhibition is removed enhancing the movement of skin from external auditory canal

REASON FOR INTERMITTENT DISCHARGE IN OTITIS MEDIA

1. Virtuous circle- Discharge & healing of perforation dictated by acute inflammatory changes

2. vicious circle - Incomplete healing predisposes the ear to further acute episodic and become chronic

3. Contaminated water entering ear, Low host immunity leads to frequent infection

4. Thickening the residual drum head with tympanosclerosis

5. Retraction pockets lose their ability to propel keratin into the self-cleaning system of the ear canal.

REASONS FOR INCREASED INCIDENCE OF ASOM IN CHILDREN

1. Wider eustachian tube than adults

2. Short and straight Eustachian tube

3. Elastin content of tissue around the ET lumen in less than in adults

4. Relative floppiness of ET in children

5. Abundance of lymphoid tissue around the ET lumen in children.

"The child's continuous crying at night is likely due to venous stasis around the ET caused by their sleeping position and reduced swallowing during the night."

CAUSES OF HEARING LOSS IN CSOM

1. Perforation of the Tympanic membrane –depends on size & position.

    a) Small Central perforation - less hearing loss,

    b) Large Central perforation- more hearing loss

2. The loss of round window baffle effect

3. Destruction of Ossicular chain or loss of stapes arch

4. presence of active mucosal disease like fibrosis, tympanosclerosis, polyp, granulation & cholesteatoma

5. cochlear damage by diffusion of the toxic products of inflammation through the scala tympani via round window membrane

CAUSES OF FAILURE OF HEALING OF A PERFORATION

1. A defect too large for Epithelium to bridge

2. Failure of the Epithelium or lamina to proliferate due to damage from trauma

3. Infection

4. Failure to remove the cause of perforation

5. Using Ear drops or Earbuds introduce the infection to squamous Epithelium around the margin.

SEQUELAE OF ASOM

1. Otitis media with effusion
2. High frequency sensorineural hearing loss
3. Persistent perforation of Tympanic membrane
4. Adhesive otitis media
5. CSOM

SEQUELAE OF OTITIS MEDIA WITH EFFUSION

(sequelae means processes that remain within the mucoperiosteum)

1. Attic erosion and Attic retraction.
2. Atrophy of pars tensa & Atelectasis
3. Tympanosclerosis & Myringosclerosis
4. Myringostapediopexy
5. Ossicular erosion

SEQUELAE OF CSOM

1. Permanent perforation syndrome
2. Healed central perforation
3. Resolution
4. Tympanosclerosis
5. Ossicular necrosis

CAUSES OF EAR CANAL WALL STENOSIS

1. Inadequate packing

2. Early removal of canal pack

3. Postoperative infection

4. Lining by respiratory Epithelium leads to mucus secretions

5. Extensive thinning of the posterior canal wall

ENZYME IN OTOSCLEROSIS

1. Alpha chymotrypsin and trypsin

2. Phosphatidic acid

3. Collagenase

4. Lactic Dehydrogenase

6. Ribonuclease

ENZYME IN CHOLESTEATOMA

1. Acid phosphatase Protease

2. IL1 alpha IL1 beta, PGEs

3. Collagenase,

4. Cathepsin k & calpain l & ll

5. TNF alpha and beta and TGF alpha & beta. Matrix metalloproteinases 2 and 9 & bone morphogenic protein.

ENZYME IN MUCOCELE

1. Prostaglandin E2

2. Interleukin-1

3. Tumor necrosis factor

4. Collagenase

5. Trypsin

HOW DO YOU MANAGE THE CASE OF CSOM

1. Examination of Ear with microscopy or Otoendoscopy.

2. Aural culture and sensitivity

3. Pure tone audiogram

4. X-ray Mastoid (Both ears)

5. Rule out septic foci using diagnostic nasal endoscopy and CT-PNS. In case of Unsafe CSOM, HRCT- temporal bone required. In case of complication, MRI BRAIN required.

9

DISEASE OF EXTERNAL EAR

CONGENITAL SYNDROME ASSOCIATED WITH MICROTIA

1. Treachercollins syndrome
2. Otomandibular syndrome of konigmark & Gorlin
3. The branchio otic dysplasia Fraser syndrome
4. LacrimoAuriculodento digital LADD syndrome
5. The oto renal genital syndrome

CONGENITAL MALFORMATIONS OF PINNA

1. Anotia, Polyotia, Macrotia and microtia
2. Bat ear or lop ear — Absence of antihelix
3. Synotia & Malotia — Ear Placed below the maxilla
4. Mozart ear — Fusion of crura of Antihelix
5. Wildermuth ear — Prominence of Antihelix

EAR FINDING IN DOWN'S SYNDROME

1. Small Pinna
2. Poorly developed lobule
3. EAC atresia with hearing loss
4. Ossicular chain defects
5. Otitis media Effusion

EAR PINNA DISEASES

1. Hematoma auris, pseudocyst of pinna
2. Perichondritis, Erysipelas
3. Sebaceous cyst, Keloid
4. Gout, Ochronosis
5. Chondrodermatitis Helicis (wrinkler's) & Relapsing polychondritis

CONGENITAL TUMORS OF EXTERNAL EAR PINNA

1. Haemangioma - Commonest Tumor
2. Capillary and cavernous hemangioma
3. Compact hemangioma
4. Lymphangioma
5. Dermoid list - near Anterior Border of Ascending Limb of helix

ACQUIRED ATRESIA OF EAC

1. Trauma
2. Simple mastoid or ear surgery
3. Keloid of EAC
4. Chronic Otitis Externa
5. Burns, Radiation and Neoplasm

PREAURICULAR SINUS

1. It occurs at Anterior margin of the Ascending limb of the helix of the external ear
2. It due to failure of fusion of First and second pharyngeal arch (Hillocks)

3. This track inwards and may follow a complex course ending blindly till tympanic ring

4. It may cause Preauricular abscess which is treated by I&D, If recurrent, wide local excision.

5. Collaural fistula open superiorly in the floor of EAC and inferiorly in the Ant border of SCM behind the Jaw

PREAURICULAR SINUS CLASSIFICATION

(Congdon's classification)

1. Pre auricular type & Postauricular type

2. Marginal helicine type & Posterior helicine type

3. Crural type

4. Helico-lobular type

6. Centrilobular type

DD OF AURAL POLYPS IN EAC

1. Arise from Middle ear cleft in case of Tubotympanic type of CSOM

2. Attic polyp seen in atticoantral type of CSOM (cholesteatoma)

3. Malignancy of EAC

4. Glomus jugulare

5. Rhabdomyosarcoma

"EAC Polyps should never be avulsed and polyps are to be cut off as close as to the base"

CLASSIFICATION OF OTITIS EXTERNA

1. Acute & Chronic

2. Localized (Furunculosis) and

-diffuse (Singapore or Tropical ear)

A] Desquamative - Raw, Red, Shiny Skin

b) Infiltrative-canal edema

3. Infective bullosa   - viral bacterial fungal and myringitis

4. Reactive   - seborrheic, eczematous, psoriasis, Lupus erythematosus and Atopic dermatitis (Besnier's)

5. Malignant otitis externa (invasive/granulomatous/ necrotizing

BENEFITS OF IG (ICHTHAMMOL & GLYCERINE) PACK FOR OTITIS EXTERNA

1. Absorbs water and decreases the tension

2. Antiseptic and bacteriostatic

3. Counter Pressure

4. Splinting action and EAC will not move with mastication

5. Local irritant thus stimulates the local circulation

MALIGNANT OTITIS EXTERNA (SKULL BASE OSTEOMYELITIS)

1. Pseudomonas infection potential to involve the EAC & skull base in Diabetics or immunocompromised patients (AIDS)

2. Local microangiopathy & Altered leukocyte function causes cellulitis and osteomyelitis in DM

3. Nubbin of granulation tissue found between junction of cartilage sand bony part tof EAC on the floor of the canal

4. Facial nerve palsy is due to extension of infection posteriorly to the stylomastoid foramen.

5. pseudomonas produces exotoxin, elastase which digest the vessel walls causing a necrotizing vasculitis

"Technetium bone scan and gallium 67 scan to assess the disease extension" and improvement of disease.

OTOMYCOSIS

1. The bacterial flora of the ear canal is lost by using topical antibiotics and when skin PH is lowered. An acidic milieu allows an overgrowth of fungus

2. Aspergillosis (black) and candidiasis (white)

3. Canal is clogged with puttaceous debris which is magenta colored studded with glistering white deposits. candidiasis has a wet blotting paper appearance

4. Pain in case of secondary Infection

5. Treated by aural toileting followed by anti-fungal drops

KERATOSIS OBTURANS

1. Generalized Hyperkeratosis of canal skin which is layered in layers which block the EAC

2. On removal canal is widened

3. No bony erosion

4. EAC keratin squamous is in lamellar pattern

5. Conservative management

EXTERNAL CANAL CHOLESTEATOMA

1. Focal hyperkeratosis of Canal

2. Canal size is normal

3. Bony erosion present

4. Random pattern of squamous keratin

5. Surgical debridement and canaloplasty

COMPACT OSTEOMA OF EAC (IVORY EXOSTOSIS)

1. Bilateral

2. Association with swimming (Surfer's ear- cold water) and trauma

3. Slow Growing with small broad base attached to the underlying bone

4. Multiple and consists of dense ivory bone (V-shape appearance)

5. More common

CANCELLOUS OSTEOMA OF EAC (CUPSLR)

1. Unilateral

2. Single

3. Rapid growth occurs at tympanosquamous suture line or tympanomastoid suture line

4. Pedunculated attachment

5. Less common

OTITIS EXTERNA (FURUNCULOSIS) OF EAC

1. Post auricular tenderness   - Diffuse

2. Displacement of pinna   - forward

3. Enlarged lymph node   - Present

4. Tragal sign   - positive

5. Mastoid X Ray   - cells are seen (cellular)

ACUTE MASTOIDITIS

1. Post auricular tenderness   - Over mastoid antrum
2. Displacement of pinna   - Forwards & downwards
3. Enlarged lymph node   - Absent
4. Tragal sign   - Negative but three finger test is positive
5. Mastoid X Ray   - Acellular or cloudy

EPITHELIAL TUMORS OF EAC

1. Hidradenoma (ceruminoma)
2. Basal cell carcinoma
3. Sebaceous Tumors
4. Malignant melanoma
5. Squamous cell carcinoma

EPITHELIAL TUMORS OF MIDDLE EAR

1. Choristoma (Salivary tissue)
2. Benign Adenoma
3. Adenocarcinoma
4. Heffner's tumor (2° from Endolymphatic Sac)
5. Squamous cell carcinoma

AETIOLOGICAL FACTORS OF EPITHELIAL TUMORS OF EAR

1. Actinic rays, trauma, frostbite
2. Psoriasis, Xeroderma pigmentosum
3. Chronic otitis media
4. Radiotherapy

5. Aflatoxins Produced by Aspergillus flavus

CONDUCTIVE HEARING LOSS AFTER RADIO-THERAPY

1. Thick mucus blocking ET opening of Nasopharynx
2. Atresia of ET
3. Necrosis of ET
4. Fibrosis of levator palati muscle
5. Middle ear Effusion

SYMPTOM & SIGNS OF EAR TUMORS

1. Painful
2. Bloodstained ear Discharge
3. Hearing loss & unsteadiness
4. Facial paralysis
5. Trismus & lower four CN paralysis

SPREADS OF EAR TUMORS

1. Laterally — parotid gland TM joint & Concha & Postauricular area
2. Medially — Middle Ear (Tympano Tubal)
3. Superiorly — Tegmen & Middle fossa (Petro mastoid)
4. Inferiorly — Jugular bulb & Lower 4 cranial nerves
5. Posteriorly — Sigmoid sinus & posterior fossa

SURGICAL TREATMENT FOR EAR TUMORS

1. Sleeve resection
2. Lateral Temporal bone resection
3. Modified temporal bone resection

4. Subtotal Petrosectomy– Transection lateral to ICA, Medial to arcuate eminence

5. Total Petrosectomy

COMPLICATION OF RT IN EAR TUMORS

1. Osteo Radio Necrosis of Bone

2. Stenosis of EAC

3. Damage to brain

4. Damage to brainstem

5. Damage to Eyes

BULLOUS MYRINGITIS

1. Myringitis bullosa haemorrhagica

2. Serous fluid containing vesicles (blebs) in the superficial layer of the Tympanic membrane.

3. Aetiology-mycoplasma influenza Virus followed by URI

4. Pain in the ear.

5. Occasionally associated with URI and cranial nerve palsy.

GRANULAR MYRINGITIS

1. Non-specific granulation tissue affecting the superficial epithelial layers of the Tympanic membrane

2. Caused by Self-cleaning ear with buds or sharp objects.

3. Granulation Extends to the skin of the meatus and a fibrotic stenosis result

4. Pain the ear.

5. Response to steroid

FOREIGN BODY IN THE EAR

1. Do not use water to remove batteries, food or plant material.

2. Use oil or alcohol for an insect

3. Oil can cause toxic to insects

4. Impact FB should remove by anesthesia

5. Ear probe, suction and ear syringe were used to remove the FB.

10

EUSTACHIAN TUBE

ANATOMY OF ET [PHARYNGOTYMPANIC TUBE]

1. It is channel connecting anterior wall of tympanic cavity and lateral wall of nasopharynx

2. 38 mm length [laterally bony 12 mm & medially cartilaginous 24 mm], runs downwards, forwards and medially from middle ear.

3. It is lined by ciliated epithelium with goblet cell and glands

4. The roof of the bony part of the tube is separated by a thin bone from the tensor tympani muscle and the carotid artery also separated by a plate of bone, lies medial to the tube.

5. The tube opens 1-1.25 cm behind and little below the posterior end of the inferior turbinate. The opening is almost triangular in shape and is surrounded above and behind by the tubal elevation. [the apex of cartilage is attached to the isthmus 2 mm of bony portion, while the wider medial end lies directly under the mucosa of the nasopharynx and form elevation.

SURGICAL IMPORTANCE OF ET

1. Behind the tubal elevation is fossa of Rosenmuller which is hind area of cancer [NPC]

2. The salpingopharyngeal fold stretches from the lower part of the tubal elevation downwards to the wall of the pharynx

3. The tensor palati muscle separates the tube from Otic ganglion, the mandibular nerve, its branches, the chorda tympani and the middle meningeal artery.

4. The Levator palati muscle first lies inferior to the tube, then crosses to the medial side and spreads out into the soft palate.

5. Tubal opening during swallowing & yawning.

NORMAL FINDING OF NASOPHARYNGEAL END OF ET WITH ENDOSCOPY (1 mm)

1. Soft palate elevation and medial rotation of posterior medial wall with posterior pharyngeal wall motion

2. Eustachian tube opening

3. Tensor Veli palatini further opening towards bony part of ET

4. Convert bulge seen resting on anterior lateral ET with Final opening

5. Passive closure of Eustachian tube.

ABNORMAL FINDING OF ENDOSCOPIC OF ET

1. No opening

2. Moderate to minimal opening

3. Mucosal edema

4. Obstructive mucosal disease

5. Decreased lateral wall motion

ETIOLOGY OF ET DYSFUNCTIONS

1. congenital anomalies   - Cleft palate & Cranio basal
2. Inflammation   - Nose, Adenoids and sinuses
3. Trauma   - ET catheterization & fracture of maxilla
4. Neoplasm   - Benign & malignant
5. ET obstruction
    1. Functional - Patulous
    2. Mechanical – infection, allergy, adenoid
    3. Palatal paralysis
    4. Post radiation
    5. Malnutrition & ciliary motility disorders.

CAUSES OF PATULOUS ET

1. Atrophic Rhinitis, senility & sudden loss of weight
2. Pregnancy
3. OCP & diuretics consuming Patients
4. Myasthenia gravis & lower motor neuron disease
5. Gasserian ganglion surgery

MUSCLES ATTACHED TO THE ET

1. Tensor veli Palatini (TVP) – Lateral & Medial bundle fibers
2. Levatorpalati - permits the action of TVP
3. Laryngopharynx
4. Tensor tympani
5. OSTMANN Fat – Submucosal seromucous gland

11

DISEASES OF MIDDLE EAR

1. ASOM

TREATMENT OF ASOM

1. 1 year baby - Watchful waiting
2. Use of Antibiotic leads to an increase in the incidence of serous otitis media
3. Adults - nothing but pain relief and no antibiotics
4. Recurrent Asom – adenoidectomy with or without myringotomy and ventilating tubes
5. Cortical mastoidectomy if complications exist

COMPLICATIONS OF ASOM

1. Facial Paralysis
2. Otogenic Intracranial Complications

    - Meningitis due to Hemophilus influenzae type B
3. Acute Mastoiditis
    1. Bezold's abscess   - behind sternomastoid muscle
    2. Citteli's Abscess   - Posterior belly of Digastric
    3. Luc's abscess   - Infratemporal region
    4. zygomatic abscess
4. Brain abscess and extradural abscess
5. Lateral sinus thrombosis

APPROACH TO PETROUS APEX ABSCESS (GRADENIGO SYNDROME)

1. Eagleton's Operation - Superior approach by removal of tegmen to base of zygoma

2. Thornvaldt's operation - superior approach along the supra labyrinthine tracts

3. Almoor's Operation - Interior approach -a space bounded by cochlea, carotid artery and tegmen tympani

4. Lempert - Ramadier operation - Between cochlea and carotid artery via Peritubal cells

5. Frenckner's Operation - Through the arch of superior semicircular canal

2. OME ETIOLOGY OF OTITIS MEDIA WITH EFFUSION

1) Due to palatal problem - cleft palate & submucous cleft palate (misdirected action of LVP muscle)

2) Due to altered mucociliary system - **IAS-HS**

   1. Infection – Streptococcus pneumoniae, Haemophilus Influenzae, Moraxella catarrhalis, streptococcus pyogenes.

   2. **Allergy** – IgE & passive smoking

   3. **Ciliary Abnormalities** - Kartagener syndrome

   4. **Immunological factor** – Secretory IgA & IgG2

   5. **Surfactant deficiency** in the Eustachian tube

   6. **Hormonal factor** – high estrogen, hypothyroidism

3) Middle ear gas composition

   1. Middle ear acts like gas pocket – high diffusion into blood

2. Chemoreceptor (Substance P & CGRP) Acts with a neural stretch receptor in the Tympanic membrane.

3. Sniff induced negative pressure

4. Antigenic stimulation

5. Cold air in the EAC leads to OME due to vagal stimulation.

4) Craniofacial abnormalities - Increase basal angle of the skull in relation to the cranial cavity

   - Down's, Hurler's, Hunter's syndrome.

   - Fragile X, Bifid uvula

5) Adenoid and the nasopharyngeal carcinoma, AIDS & Barotrauma & RT.

3. CSOM

General Aetiology of COM

1. Environmental - Low socio-economic status, Overcrowding home

2. Genetic - Small mastoid air cell

3. Infection - Mono infection, mixed anaerobes & No growth

4. URI & previous otitis media

5. Auto immunity & Allergy with ET malfunction

MEDICAL TREATMENT TO STOP THE EAR DISCHARGE (CSOM)

1. Aural toileting - dry mopping, wet mopping & suction clearance

2. Local antibiotic drops (Topical)

3. Systemic Antibiotics

4. NSAID

5. Nasal decongestants and Antihistamines.

FINDINGS OF COALESCENT MASTOIDITIS

1. Continuous purulent Ear discharge more than 2 weeks

2. Mastoid tenderness & thickening of periosteum

3. Sagging of posterosuperior wall of external auditory canal due to Periosteal thickening adjacent to antrum

4. Nipple like protrusion seen through Tympanic membrane perforation

5. Subperiosteal abscess with displacement of auricle.

TYPE OF CENTRAL PERFORATION

1. Pinhole perforation- ASOM

2. Small CP- one quadrant less than 25% of pars tensa

3. Large CP- Two quadrant less than 50%

4. Subtotal perforation- Three quadrant less than 75%

5. Total perforation – Tympanic annulus involved 100%

CAUTERIZATION ROLE IN CENTRAL PERFORATION

1. Central Perforation of Tympanic membrane less than 65% size

2. Dry ear for at least 6 weeks

3. Wide external auditory canal

4. Patient ready for weekly visits

5. Traumatic Perforation

HEALING OF PERFORATION BY CAUTERY

1. 20% Silver nitrate (Ag No3) or 50% Trichloroacetic Acid (using cotton)

2. Applicator is stroked over the edge of perforation in an inward to outward fashion to break the epithelial barrier

3. Repetition of cautery every week until we see a new pink, actively growing margin seen.

4. Rim of the perforation should be kept moist

5. Tympanic membrane closes in all three layers unlike the spontaneous healing which heals by two layers.

CHOLESTEATOMA

Types of the Cholesteatoma (Johannes Mueller coined the term 1829)

1. Extradural Cholesteatoma - Petrous

2. Intradural cholesteatoma - Cerebellopontine angle

3. Congenital cholesteatoma - Jugular fossa, middle ear, petrous & cerebellopontine angle

4. Primary Acquired cholesteatoma -

   a) Posterior Epitympanic

   b) Anterior epitympanic &

   c) posterior-superior mesotympanic

5. Secondary Acquired cholesteatoma [Lillie type III)- Sinus cholesteatoma (Pars tensa cholesteatoma)

CHARACTERISTICS OF CONGENITAL CHOLESTEATOMA

1. Location limited to the Anterosuperior quadrant in 77%

2. Encapsulation

3. White retro tympanic mass with intact TM

4. Translucent drum moves independently from the white retro tympanic mass

5. Normal pars tensa & pars flaccida.

HYPOTHESIS OF DEVELOPMENT OF CHOLESTEATOMA

1. Negative pressure or invagination-(Wittmack) Retraction pocket in attic followed serous otitis media

2. Invasion I or epithelial immigration-

   Acute otitis media causes attic perforation – Squamous growth into middle ear

3. Invasion II- Migration of squamous Epithelium into retraction pockets (Habermann, Weiss Jackson & Lim)

4. Metaplasia I or Implantation-Squamous Epithelium forms into cyst.

5. Metaplasia II [Wendt] - Chronic otitis media irritates the Squamous Epithelium and leads to hypertrophy proliferation (Reudi). -Basal cell hyperplasia (Langer)

THEORIES OF BONE DESTRUCTION BY CHOLESTEATOMA

1. Pressure theory - Normal Capillary pressure 25 mmHg doesn't cause any necrosis

2. Pyogenic osteitis theory – Pseudomonas aeruginosa, B. Fragilis, Proteus, E.Coli Fusobacterium

3. Enzymatic theory (Lautenschlager)

   -N Acetyl –B Hexosaminidase & Matrix Metalloproteinase

   -TNF alpha – Stimulates osteoclasts

4. chemical activity and bone resorption - Hydroxyapatite $\downarrow$PH

5. Role of Nitrous Oxide

DERLACKI & CLEMIS CRITERIA OF CONGENITAL CHOLESTEATOMA (1965)

1. Development behind an intact tympanic membrane

2. No previous history of otitis media

3. An origin from embryonal inclusion of squamous epithelium

4. From undifferentiated epithelium

5. Which changes into Squamous Epithelium during development

LEVENSON CRITERIA OF CONGENITAL CHOLESTEATOMA

1. A white mass medial to a normal Tympanic membrane

2. Normal Pars flaccida and pars tensa

3. No prior history of otorrhea or preformation or otological procedures

4. Canal atresia and intramembranous & Giant cholesteatoma

5. Prior bouts of otitis media are not grounds for exclusion as congenital disease (Levenson added that the presence of uncomplicated acute otitis media does not exclude congenital cholesteatoma).

SPREAD OF CHOLESTEATOMA

1. Posterior spread of posterior Epitympanic Cholesteatoma from the Prussack's space to Superior incudal space spread lateral to Incus to Aditus Antrum

2. Inferior spread of posterior Epitympanic Cholesteatoma from Prussack's space via Posterior pouch of Von Troeltsch to Posterior mesotympanum to Stapes, Sinus Tympani & Facial recess

3. Anterior spread of posterior epitympanic cholesteatoma from Prussack's space spread Anterior to malleolus to Anterior Epitympanum spread to Supratubal recess & Anterior mesotympanum via anterior pouch of Von Troeltsch

4. Posterior Mesotympanic cholesteatoma from Sinus tympani spread to inferior incudal space spread medial to incus via posterior tympanic isthmus to aditus & antrum.

5. Anterior Epitympanic Cholesteatoma Supratubal recess spread to anterior pouch of Von Troeltsch

SIGNS OF CHOLESTEATOMA

1. Foul smelling ear discharge due to osteitis & saprophytic

2. Continue ear discharge due to shedding of squamous

3. Blood stains ear discharge due to granulation

4. Hearing loss or cholesteatoma hearing

5. Cholesteatoma flacks -pearly white with fishy odor, these flakes are reappear after cleaning, whereas Otomycosis flacks don't reappear after cleaning

COMPLICATION OF CSOM - ROUTE OF SPREAD

1. Through bone by infection or cholesteatoma

2. Through infected clot within small veins.   -to cerebellum via Lateral sinus

   -to temporal lobe via superior petrosal sinus

-to Brain abscess via periarteriolar spaces of Virchow Robin.

3. Through normal anatomical pathways

    1. RW, OW

    2. Aqueduct of cochlear and vestibular

    3. Dehisce of jugular bulb

    4. Tegmen

    5. suture line of temporal bone.

4. Through non- anatomical bony defects - Trauma, surgery & Neoplastic erosion.

5. Through surgical defects - stapedotomy & LSC fenestration.

COMPLICATION OF CSOM [complication means processes that occur outside the mucoperiosteum of middle ear cleft)

THE PROPENSITY FOR SPREAD OF INFECTION DEPENDS ON

1. Age

2. Immunization Status, diabetes mellitus, Leukemia

3. Virulence of organism - streptococcus pneumonia type III, H-influenzae type B

4. Susceptibility to chemotherapeutic elimination

5. Efficacy of treatment of the underlying middle ear Disease

COMPLICATION OF COM

A. **Intra Temporal complication**

1) Middle ear complications – Facial palsy, Ossicular lesion & Central perforation

2) Inner ear complication - labyrinthitis, Petrositis & sensorineural hearing loss

3) Mastoid Complication – Coalescent Mastoiditis

B. **Extra temporal**

4) Extra temporal intracranial Complication

    a) Extradural subdural lesions and brain abscess

    b) Lateral sinus thrombosis

    c) Otitis hydrocephalus

    d) Meningitis

    e) Tetanus

5) Extra temporal Extra cranial Complication

    a) Bezold's abscess

    b) Citelle's abscess

    c) LUC's Abscess

    d) Zygomatic abscess

    e) Subperiosteal abscess

TYPES OF LABYRINTHITIS

1) Purulent labyrinthitis – Tympanogenic, Menigogenic & Tuberculous

2) Non purulent diffuse serous labyrinthitis – diplacusis

Non-Purulent diffuse suppurative Labyrinthitis – Acute and chronic

3) Circumscribed labyrinthitis - Inflammation Restricted to a discrete portion of labyrinth and Endosteum.

4) Peri labyrinthitis - Fistula by mastoid surgery with normal vestibular function

5) Para labyrinthitis - Vestibular irritation by inflammatory disease of Endosteum

OTOGENIC EXTRADURAL ABSCESS (Middle fossa Extradural abscess)

1. Commonest of all intracranial complications arising from middle ear infection

2. Dura is tough and resistant to invasion and destruction, so there is collection of Pus between bone & dura matter

3. This abscess is confined to the upper surface of tegmen tympani & lateral to arcuate eminence. Due to attachment of the dura to the arcuate eminence, it impedes the development of a large volume of Pus. This Abscess may develop medial to arcuate eminence over the petrous apex causing Gradenigo's syndrome

4. Erosion Through the skull to the exterior would produce subperiosteal abscess. "Pott's puffy tumor"

5. Posterior fossa extradural abscess limited by attachment of dura laterally to sigmoid sinus, medially to internal auditory canal & subarcuate fossa leads to perisinus abscess & involve jugular vein.

SUBDURAL ABSCESS – STREP. MILLERI

1. The granulation tissue inflammatory reactions tend to obliterate the spaces

2. This granulation tissue converted to fibrous tissue Leads to necrosis of the dura, pus collected between dura and arachnoid

3. Seropurulent effusion becomes frankly purulent - SOL

4. Cortical thrombophlebitis leads to multiple small abscesses

5. ubdural PUS tends to accumulate near the falx cerebri at tentorium cerebelli

LATERAL SINUS THROMBOPHLEBITIS (LATERAL SINUS = SIGMOID SINUS + TRANSVERSE SINUS)

1. Mural thrombus formed from extradural perisinus abscess and release infected clot after it breaks, released into systemic circulation causing bacteremia, septicemia & septic venous embolization

2. Propagation of the thrombin upwards to Torcula Herophili and downwards to internal jugular vein to subclavian vein

3. Otalgia neck, pain with mastoid tenderness and stiffness along the sterno mastoid muscle with fever

4. a) Picket-fence pattern fever -> fever was high & swinging rigors with profuse sweating at 39-40°c and then fever falls

   b) Griesinger sign -> pitting edema over the occipital region well behind the mastoid process caused by a clot within a large mastoid emissary vein

   c) Lillie crow's sign -> When one sinus is occluded by thrombus, digital compression of the opposite jugular will produce dilation of retinal veins on normal side

   d) Queckenstedt test or Tobe Ayer test -> pressure over the internal jugular vein in case of thrombosis there is no or very slow rise of 10-20 mmHg of CSF pressure. (Normal rise is around 50-100 mmhg)

   e) Delta sign -> filling defects in sinus with enhancement due to increased density of the fresh clot. This empty triangle sign seen in CT-Scan

5. The thrombosed sinus wall feels firm with opaque & absence of bleed on needle whereas normal sinus is soft, bluish & compressible with blunt probe, bleeds on the needle.

OTOGENIC BRAIN ABSCESS

1. Temporal bone abscess usually occupies the middle third of the temporal lobe and this abscess spreads via osteitic tegmen tympani or Virchow Robin spaces

2. Cerebellar abscess occupies the anterior part of the lateral lobe of the cerebellum and this abscess developed from Trautman's triangle or lateral sinus thrombophlebitis

3. Cerebral - temporo sphenoidal abscess - nominal aphasia, Quadratic homonymous hemianopia when the abscess extends superficially the face is first affected then the arm & the leg, but if the abscess spread inwards towards the posterior part of the internal capsule the order of paralysis is reversed, the leg is affected first then the arm and lastly the face

4. Pathology in areas of cerebral edema or encephalitis leads to formation of capsule and central part liquefies the abscess leading to rupture

5. Clinical stages are stages of encephalitis (1-3 days) stages of latency (4-10 days), stage of enlarging abscess (10-13 day) & terminal stage (14 days)

OTITIC HYDROCEPHALUS [SYMONDS SYNDROME)

1. Lateral sinus obstructions by thrombus or thrombosis extends into Superior sagittal Sinus impedes CSF resorption by pacchionian bodies

2. Idiopathic benign intracranial hypertension

3. Higher incidence of sinus thrombosis in right side over left side due to variation of venous arrangement in the skull

4. Headache drowsiness blurred vision & lateral rectus palsy

5. Most common is children & Adolescents

CAUSES OF FISTULA IN LABYRINTH

1. Surgical

2. Cholesteatoma

3. Syphilis & Tuberculosis

4. Neoplastic ear disease & glomus

5. arotrauma

TREATMENT OF LABYRINTHINE FISTULA

1. A slight change in color at the junction of the matrix and subjacent bone suggests a possible fistula

2. Matrix should be removed from other sites first, then dissection carried out slowly under high power magnification

3. The operations are to remove the matrix, or to leave Matrix in place of fistula

4. If it is an open cavity (radical mastoidectomy) Matrix over fistula left undisturbed or matrix is completely removed from the fistula, the defect should be closed with fascia or perichondrium & fibrin glue

5. If it is an intact canal wall technique, any fistula matrix can be left in its place. The patient is called for a second sitting after a month, by that time the abandoned matrix

will be formed by small epithelial cells which can easily
be removed.

CAUSES OF VERTIGO AFTER MASTOID SURGERY

1. Unrelated vestibular disease

2. Persistent middle ear diseases Peri Labyrinthitis

3. Delayed Endolymphatic hydrops & Breakdown of central compensation affecting labyrinthine function

4. Cerebellar Abscess

5. Vestibular neuroma after labyrinthectomy

UNILATERAL LABYRINTHINE DESTRUCTION EFFECTS [RIGHT SIDE]

1. Right side skew deviation of the eyes

2. Flexion of the Neck &

3. Rotation of the occiput to Right side

4. Spontaneous Nystagmus to Left side

5. Increased extensor tone in the limbs of left side

BILATERAL LABYRINTHINE DESTRUCTION EFFECTS "ZERO MAN"

1. Severe loss of tone in all postural muscles

2. Severe degrees of imbalance ataxia

3. No nystagmus or vertigo

4. Underwater disorientation is complete

5. Without aid of sight, patient cannot stand

TYMPANOPLASTY

Types of Tympanoplasty

1. I   - Graft rests on malleus
2. II   - Graft rests on incus
3. III   - Graft Rests on stapes head
4. IV   - Graft rests on mobile stapes footplate
5. V   - Graft rests on LSC if Stapes fixed

    VI   - Sono inversion Graft placed on RW leave OW exposed

TYPES OF TYMPANOPLASTY (FARRIOR CLASSIFICATION)

1. I - Reconstruction of New Tympanic membrane. All ossicles are intact.

2. II - Reconstruction of New Tympanic membrane in its natural position.

3. III - Reconstruction of New Tympanic membrane on top of mobile stapes head

   Type II IG (incus graft), IGM (incus malleus graft), MG (malleus graft), BG (bone graft), PORP [partial ossicular reconstruction prosthesis)

4. IV - Reconstruction of new Tympanic membrane on the footplate of stapes

   type IV IG, MG, BG, CG, TORP (Total ossicular reconstruction prosthesis)

5. V- Reconstruction of New Tympanic membrane over fistula of semicircular canal. Type V a Lateral semicircular canal

   Type V b stapedectomy

AUSTIN'S CLASSIFICATION OF OSSICULAR CHAIN DEFECT

1. Incus absent + malleus handle & stapes head present
2. Incus absent + malleus handle absent + stapes head present
3. Incus absent + malleus handle present + stapes head absent
4. Incus absent + malleus handle absent + stapes head absent
5. Isolated loss of stapes head is very rare.

    ->Pennington Type Ia & Ib -Vertical malleus/stapes assembly

    Type II – Horizontal Malleus/Stapes Assembly

    ->Wehrs

    Type I – Notched incus with short process

    Type II – Notched incus with long process

OSSICULAR BONE AUTOGRAFTS

1. Interposed ossicles (short process of incus or sculptured malleus)
2. Transposition of ossicle (Incus remnant)
3. Tympanum Malleus Stapediopexy
4. Merits are vascularization of marrows space, Viable osteocytes in Lacunae but no new bone formation
5. Demerits are Ankylosis, Occult osteitis and Evidence of erosion macroscopically, So Ossicles with Adherent Squamous Epithelium or Cholesteatoma should never be used in reconstruction

OSSICULOPLASTY PRINCIPLES LIKE (TRACS)=

1. TENSION,
2. REBOUNDING,
3. ANGULATION,
4. CENTRING and
5. SPACING

(Taking an autograft ossicular prosthesis is crafting art. Bone over sinodural angle is preferred site because of its thickness)

CLASSIFICATION OF CARTILAGE TYMPANOPLASTY METHODS (TOS 2008).

1. Group A:

Cartilage tympanoplasty with palisades,

strips, and slices.

1. Cartilage palisades in underlay tympanoplasty techniques.
2. Cartilage palisades in on-lay tympanoplasty techniques.
3. Tympanoplasty with broad cartilage palisades.
4. Cartilage strips in underlay tympanoplasty techniques.
6. Cartilage strips in on-lay tympanoplasty techniques.
7. The Dornhoffer underlay cartilage slice mosaic tympanoplasty.

2. Group B:

8. Cartilage tympanoplasty with foils, thin plates, and thick plates
9. Underlay tympanoplasty with cartilage foils and thin plates.
10. On-lay tympanoplasty with cartilage foils and thin

plates.

11. On-lay tympanoplasty with thick cartilage plates.

12. Underlay tympanoplasty with thick cartilage plates.

3. Group C:

13. Tympanoplasty with cartilage-perichondrium composite island grafts

14. Superior (attic) cartilage-perichondrium island graft tympanoplasty.

15. Posterior cartilage-perichondrium composite island graft tympanoplasty.

16. Superior and posterior cartilage-perichondrium composite island graft tympanoplasty.

17. Total pars tensa cartilage-perichondrium composite

4. Group D:

Tympanoplasty with special total pars tensa cartilage-perichondrium composite grafts

18. Annular cartilage-perichondrium composite graft tympanoplasty.

19. "Crown cork" cartilage-perichondrium composite graft tympanoplasty.

20. Cartilage shield T-tube tympanoplasty.

5. Group E:

Cartilage-perichondrium composite island graft tympanoplasty for anterior, inferior, and subtotal perforations.

21. Underlay tympanoplasty techniques with cartilage-perichondrium composite island graft.

22. In-lay underlay tympanoplasty techniques with cartilage-perichondrium composite island graft.

23. On-lay tympanoplasty techniques with cartilage-perichondrium composite island graft.

24. In-lay on-lay tympanoplasty techniques with cartilage-perichondrium composite island graft

Group F:

Special cartilage tympanoplasty methods

25. In-lay butterfly cartilage tympanoplasty

26. Composite chondro perichondrial clip tympanoplasty: The triple "C" technique.

12

GRAFTS USED IN THE EAR SURGERY

GRAFTS IN EAR SURGERY (TYMPANOPLASTY, MASTOIDECTOMY)

1. Autografts-Temporalis Fascia, Tragal Perichondrium
   -Tragal cartilage, fat, vein, fascia lata & skin

2. Allografts (homograft) - Dura mater, Tympanomeatal Graft

3. Xenograft(heterograft) - bovine jugular vein and calf Cecal serosa

4. Orthotopic Graft - Tympano Ossicular allografts from Cadaver

   within 12 hrs of death)

5. Heterotopic graft - Septal cartilage allograft

ADVANTAGES OF TEMPORALIS FASCIA

"Thinner the graft better the result thicker the graft better the take up"

1. Good Survival

2. Low metabolic rate

3. Readily available

4. Thickness of Graft same as tympanic membrane

5. Close to operating site

ADVANTAGES OF CARTILAGE GRAFT (JOHN L. DORNHOFLER)

1. Hearing results with cartilage has no difference than that of fascia graft

2. Cartilage is well tolerated by middle ear & long-term survival

3. Cartilages are nourished largely by diffusion and become well incorporated with Tympanic membrane

4. Cartilage retains its (3 R') Rigid quality and Resists resorption and Retraction (prevent) of Tympanic membrane

5. Softening occurs when the time matrix of the cartilage remains intact but Empty lacunae and degeneration of the chondrocytes occur. Hence, the thickness of cartilage grafts is reduced.

PRESERVATION OF ALLOGRAFT

1. 70% ethyl alcohol at +/- 3 degree Celsius

2. 0.02% Aqueous cialit 1 in 5000

3. 4% buffered formaldehyde fixation and 0.05% Cialit

4. 0.5% buffered glutaraldehyde and 0.02% Cialit

5. freeze-drying and Ethylene oxide gas sterilization

BIOMATERIALS

1. Bio tolerant Metals -Stainless steel, Titanium & Platinum

2. Bio Tolerant polymers a) Solid - Teflon, Silastic

   b) Porous- Proplast 1&2, Plastipore and Polycel

   c) Carbon - Carbon

3. Bio inert Aluminum Oxide ceramic-Frialit, Macor and Bioceram

4. Bio Reactive glass ceramic - Bioglass and ceravital

5. Bio Active Calcium phosphate ceramics - hydroxyapa-tite

   Tricalcium phosphate, + Fibrin glue

   "Used in PORP, TORP, Canal wall prosthesis and mastoid obliteration."

   "Ionogran"-Glass Ionomer cement (Calcium Aluminosilicates glass + unsaturated carboxylic acids)

13

FACIAL NERVE

SYNDROME ASSOCIATED WITH FACIAL NERVE DISORDER

1. Opercular syndrome, Meige's syndrome, Miehlke Syndrome

2. Weber's & Millard Gubler syndrome

3. Foville's & Moebius syndrome

4. Ramsay Hunt & Melkersson Rosenthal syndrome

5. Heerfordts's Guillain Barre syndrome

SURGICAL LANDMARK OF FACIAL NERVE

1. The facial nerve is Lateral to

   1) Ampullary end of posterior semicircular canals

   2) Pyramidal Process

2. Medial to
   1) Short process of incus

   2) Lateral semicircular canal

   3) Sinus tympani

   4) Epitympanic recess

   5) Facial ridge

3. Anterior to
   1) Lateral semicircular canal

   2) Tympanomastoid suture

   3) Digastric ridge

   4) Sigmoid sinus

4. Posterior to   1) Chorda tympani

2) Processus cochleariformis [posterosuperior]

3) Stapes

5. Superior to   1) Oval window

ALTERED FUNCTION OF VII N FOLLOWING INJURY

1. Hemifacial spasm - facial hyperkinesis

2. Synkinesis

3. Crocodile tears - faulty regeneration of fascial parasympathetic fibers

4. Stapedius tendon contraction - faulty regeneration of VII nerve

5. Facial myokymia- "bag of worms"

FACIAL NERVE INJURY

[Sunderland]   [Seddone]   [House & Brakman]

1. I   - Neuropraxia   - Grade I

2. II   - Axonotmesis   - Grade II

3. III   - Neurotmesis   - Grade III-IV

4. IV   - Partial transection - Grade IV

5. V   - Complete transection   - Grade V

BELL'S PALSY FINDING

1. Loss or decrease in ipsilateral stapedial reflex 90%

2. Viral prodrome 60%

3. Red chorda tympani 40%

4. Numbness or pain of ear, face, neck or tongue 50%

5. Positive family history 14%

MELKERSSON-ROSENTHAL SYNDROME

1. Recurrent alternating facial palsy

2. Fissured tongue

3. Labial- periorbital facial edema

4. Non-Specific Labial granuloma

5. Positive family history

BILATERAL SIMULTANEOUS FACIAL PALSY (GTPS MMC BILL)

1. Guillain - Barre syndrome and Moebius syndrome

2. Trauma & Acute Porphyria

3. Sarcoidosis & myotonic dystrophy

4. Cytomegalovirus, Botulism& Bell's palsy due to Herpes simplex

5. Infectious mononucleosis and Lyme disease

SPECIAL DIAGNOSTIC TEST FOR FACIAL PALSY

1. Schirmer test

2. Taste, Submandibular flow, Hearing & Balance test

3. Stapes reflex

4. Maximal stimulation test – 1 mA to 5 mA current

5. ENOG & EMG

ROLL OF DECOMPRESSIONS IN IDIOPATHIC PALSY (MARSH AND COKER 1991)

1. EEMG (ENOG) greater that 90% of normal

2. Paralysis of less than 21 days duration

3. No Evidence of neuropraxia deblocking on EMG

4. Age less than 60 years

5. Acceptable anesthetic risk & informed consent

SPONTANEOUS RECOVERY IN VII PALSY IS FAVORABLE

1. Response to Electrical stimulation in maintained beyond 10 days

2. Voluntary motor unit action potentials on EMG persist or return within 14 days

3. Visible facial movements in maintained or begin to appear within 3 weeks

4. Recovery can be expected within 4-6 months after parotid surgery, the surgeon can be sure that the nerve has not been disrupted

5. Incomplete or delayed onset of Facial paralysis following temporal bone #

METHOD AND TIME OF SURGERY IN VII PALSY

1. Trauma -> after 10 days - Decompression

2. Temporal bone # Incomplete or delayed palsy calls for conservative management.-exploratory surgery for complete paralysis (before 30 days because onset of fibrosis)

3. Mastoid surgery -> Before the sun sets (wait for local anesthesia elimination till 4 hrs)

4. Bell's palsy-> After 21 days

5. Facial Schwannoma, glomus etc.

Nerve suture by Millesi technique of interfascicular repair using 10-0 monofilament after freshening the proximal and distal ends of the nerve and placing an interposition graft with suture.

-Nerve grafting

10 cm - cervical cutaneous nerve

10-20 cm - Greater Auricular nerve

30-40 cm – Sural nerve

-more than 6 month

-facial reanimation

- more than 2 years - Temporalis muscle transposition

-When Nerve continuity can't restore -> XII - VII jump graft

STEPS OF FACIAL NERVE DECOMPRESSION

1. Cortical mastoidectomy - posterior tympanotomy

2. Disarticulate the incus

3. Tympanic part decompression done (thin bone lift off from facial epineurium)

4. Vertical part decompression done

5. Slitting the nerve sheath vertically on its posterior aspect with a disposable beaver knife

14

ACOUSTIC TUMOR

VESTIBULAR SCHWANNOMA

1. It arises from glial neurilemmal (Schwann cell) Junction (Obersteiner - Redlich zone) at Internal auditory canal of Superior vestibular nerve or inferior vestibular nerve

2. The tumor expands in medial direction, it invaginates arachnoid and creates a double layer and it produces a presser effect on metal blood vessels & nerves. The facial nerve is motor, (usually, the motor nerve more resistant to tumor pressure than sensory nerve), so least affected by tumor.

3. Growth of schwannoma is approx 2 mm in 1 year, and is much higher in younger Patients & recurrence tumor has 3 mm growth / 1 year

4. Hearing loss is due to pressure Effect of vessels that lead to degeneration of cochlea, loss of spiral ganglion and vacuolization of stria vascularis.

5. It is firmly encapsulated with a nodular surface. Grey, yellow & purplish mass. It has Antoni A (Palisading Pattern with large nuclei) & Antoni B [Reticular Pattern without nuclei and with verocay bodies) cells.

CLINICAL PRESENTATION OF VESTIBULAR SCHWANNOMA

1. Otological stage (<2 cm) a) Deafness   - progressive or sudden SNHL

                b) Tinnitus   - NonPulsatile

c) Imbalance - Gradually compensated

d) Facial Nerve - Altered lacrimation
(nervus intermedius)

- cachoguesia
- Defective nasolacrimal reflex
- Positive Histelbergs sign

[hypo anesthesia of posterior meatal wall)

2. Trigeminal stage (2 cm-2.5 cm) extends upwards -> - Loss of corneal sensation

-Dry eye or irritating eye

-Pain or tingling, numbness over face

-Altered thermal sensation on face & tip of tongue

3. brainstem and cerebellar compression stage->   -ataxia

-dysmetria

-dyssynergia -dysdiadochokinesia

-gait disturbances -intentional tremors

-Direction changing nystagmus (burn's) &

-Lower cranial nerve 9,10,11 palsy

4. increasing intracranial pressure -stage IV>

- Headache,

- Vomiting,

- Nausea,

- Titubation,

- Papilledema

5. Terminal stage V   - Failure of vital centers

BERA FINDINGS IN VESTIBULAR SCHWANNOMA (FIRST 7 MS)

1. Prolonged wave V absolute Latency

2. Increase Interpeak latency [normal- 0.2 ms)

3. Prolonged I to V peak (normal- 4 ms)

4. Abnormal amplitude ratio <0.5

5. Abnormal wave V prolongation

STEREOTACTIC RADIOSURGERY

1) Gamma knife in 1951 by Leksell in Stockholms

2) 201 cobalt - 60 sources of Ionizing radiation in one 20-minute session to the tumor, the location of which has been precisely identified stereotactically. The dose delivered to the center of the tumor is 15-25 Gy and to the periphery 10-15 Gy

3) Gamma knife is not total destruction of the tumor but long-term arrest of growth

4) it is used in intracranial tumor <2.5 Cm, inoperable Patients who can be discharged within 24 hrs with 96% success

5) Complication- headache, vomiting, hearing loss and facial, spinal accessory and Trigeminal neuropathy

CUSA – 1976

1) Cavitron ultrasonic surgical aspirator fragments tissue by high frequency vibration of a Titanium tip

2) The HF oscillation of the tip is desired from the ultrasonic generator within the console which provides current to a piezoelectric. Electrical energy is converted to mechanical motion at the rate of 13 to 35 Hz.

3) Tissue rupturing effect by vacuum & cavitation

4) The action is influenced by tissue water content &it's sensitivity to the vibration process. Therefore, tissue such as fat, mucous membrane, CNS parenchyma will rupture more easily than nerve & blood vessels which are rich in elastin and collagen.

5) CAVI PULSE& CUSA CEM Options are available

15

DEAFNESS

INTERMEDIATE FILAMENTS (PROTEIN DIFFER FROM ACTIN, MYOSIN & TUBULINS)

1. Cytokeratins (5,8,18,19)- Epithelial cells with Desmosomes, present in Human cochlea

2. Desmin - smooth muscle, cardiac muscle & muscle coat of vessels

3. Glial - Astrocytes & Bergmann Glial cells

4. Neurofilaments - Neurons of cervical Peripheral nerves

5. Vimentin - Mesenchymal cells

PATHOGENESIS OF CONGENITAL DEAFNESS [ORMEROD (1960)]

1. Failure to develop or interruption of genetic or toxic factor caused by maternal illness during first 3 months of pregnancy (aplasia)

2. Interruption of development

3. Degeneration of cochlea duct

4. Degeneration of Sensory End organs

5. Degeneration of nerve element

   3,4,5-Abiotrophy)

APLASIA OF INNER EAR TYPES -SCHOKNECHT 1967 (ASOM)

1. Alexander - membranous cochlear aplasia

2. Scheibe - cochlear saccular aplasia - most common

3. Mondini- incomplete development of Bony and membranous labyrinth

4. **Michel** – complete labyrinthine aplasia

5. Bing **siebenmann** type

HEREDODEGENERATIVE TYPES - ABIOTROPHY SYNDROME

1. Occurring alone in infants or in adults

2. Down's syndrome - Trisomy - shortened cochlea

3. Ectodermal – Wardenberg, Usher's & Cogan's

4. Mesodermal - Allports, Jervell - Lange Nielsen, Pendred, Hitler's & Marfan.

5. Neuroectodermal - Von Recklinghausen's, Refsum's Jamaican

HEARING LOSS DUE TO PHYSICAL AGENTS

1. Mechanoacoustical	-	Blast, Noise, Vibration
2. Electromagnetic	-	Shock, Radiation
3. Thermal	-	Cryosurgery & ultrasound

4. Head injury

5. CHL & SNHL due to blood clot, CSF, injury to ossicles, temporal bone fracture and brain damage

MIXED DEAFNESS (MIB LOW)

1. **Branchio-Oto-Renal (ear pits) At birth- congenital**

2. **Otosclerosis**

3. Langerhans cells histiocytosis

4. Mucopolysaccharidosis – children

5. Infection – ASOM, CSOM - acquired SOM

RETRO COCHLEAR DEAFNESS (MMA VFX C)

1. Meningitis, Multiple sclerosis, Medulloblastoma

2. Amyotrophic sclerosis, Friedreich ataxia

3. Xeroderma Pigmentosum

4. VKH Syndrome

5. CPA tumor – Schwannoma, Carcinomatous neuropathy

FLUCTUATING DEAFNESS (MMC LPG)

1. Meniere's

2. Metabolic SNHL (Hypoglycemia, Hypothyroidism & Hyperlipoproteinemia)

3. Cogan's (crying deafness), Cervicogenic SNHL

4. **Lermoyez**, Labyrinthine fistula & Perilymph fistula

5. Glue Ear, Glomus & HIV

ASYMMETRICAL B/L SNHL (MISS)

1. Meniere's Disease

2. Injury - Explosive, Weapon &

3. Head Injury

4. Schwannoma B/L

5. Syphilis - Congenital or late

SYMMETRICAL B/L SNHL - (PNS -MO)

1. **Presbycusis**
2. Noise induced deafness
3. Syndrome deafness (Dish – Shaped Audiogram)
4. Metabolic Deafness
5. Ototoxic Drugs (Salicylate deafness – Flat-fish audiogram curve)

UNILATERAL SNHL

1. Trauma
2. Iatrogenic by surgery
3. Mumps
4. Vestibular Schwannoma
5. Peri lymphatic Leak

SUDDEN DEAFNESS

1.	Idiopathic SNHL	- 3 day, 30 dB, 3 frequency
2.	Central Psychogenic	- Diffuse cortical encephalitis &
3.	Retro cochlear	- MMA VFX C
4.	Traumatic	- stapes fracture & perilymph fistula –
5.	Cochlear	- 1) Post meningitis measles, mumps
		2) Congenital syphilis, Rickettsia
		3) Suppurative labyrinthitis, Meniere's

     4) Profound anemia &
      ototoxicity

     5) Following spinal anesthesia
      & vascular

OTHERS DEAFNESS

1. Psychogenic   - Hysterical
2. Malingering   - feigned hearing loss
3. Immune SNHL
4. Idiopathic SNHL
   I – without URI
   II - with URI
   III – Postnatal viral labyrinthitis
5. Deafness with normal PTA - (Obscure Auditory disorders)-

  -Multiple sclerosis

  -pressure on the central auditory pathway by a tumor causes neurosis

CENTRAL DEAFNESS

1. Alzheimer disease
2. Cortical encephalitis
3. Lacunar syndrome
4. Bilateral temporal lobe damage
5. Genetic

GENETIC DEAFNESS

1. Monogenic – syndromic and non-syndromic

AD [LBWTNS]   - Leopard, Branchio-Oto-renal syndrome, Waardenberg Treacher-Collins, NF II, Stickler

AR [UPJ]   - Usher, Pendred`s, Jervell-Lange-Nielsen syndrome

2. XL   - Alport`s & Oto-Palato- Digital syndrome

3. single gene [CASO - **Crouzon`s, Apert`s, Saethre-** Chotzen-Ptosis and **Osteogenesis** imperfecta

4. Chromosomal   - Down`s syndrome

5. Heterogenous   - Goldenhar and Klippel-Feil syndrome

COCHLEAR DEAFNESS

1. Congenital Genetic at Birth

    1) Aplasia of inner ear (ASOM) - **Michel, Mondini, Scheibe, Alexander & Bing** – **Sieberman**

    2) Autosomal dominant. (LBW TNS) - Leopard, Branchio- oto-renal Waardenburg, Treacher -collins, NF-II and Stickler

    3) Autosomal recessive (UP JK) - Usher, Pendred's, Jervell- Lange Nielsen

    4) Single gene disorder (CASO) - Crouzon's, Apert's, Saethre- Chotzen, Osteogenesis imperfecta

    5) Heterogenous - Goldenhar, Klippel – Feil syndrome

    6) X-LINKED -Alport's, Oto-palato-digital

2. At childhood (N-CARR)

    1. **Norrie's**

    2. **Cogan** – crying deafness

    3. **Alport's**

    4. **Refsum's**

5. Renal tubular acidosis

3. Non-genetic - TORCH, ototoxicity, Radiotherapy, Maternal DM, Fetal Alcohol syndrome, USG

4. Perinatal - Hypoxia, Hyperbilirubinemia Preterm, LBW

5. Acquired cochlear deafness - VITAMINS-OH

ACQUIRED COCHLEAR DEAFNESS (VITAMINS –OH)

1.	Vascular causes	- HT, Burgers, Hyper coagulation & TAO
2.	a] Infection	- ASOM, Typhoid, Syphilis, Mycoplasma, Brucellosis, chlamydia, Rickettsia, & Borrelia (Lyme)
	b] Inflammatory	- Mumps, measles, EBV, pox, AIDS, Lassa fever Toxoplasmosis
3.	Traumatic	- electricity, iatrogenic, Radiotherapy, Post operative Anesthesia [N2O & Spinal) Sudden deafness after Dental Surgery.

4. Autoimmune -SLE, Systemic vasculitis, Cogan's, Polyarteritis nodosa & Relapsing polychondritis Giant cell arteritis, Kawasaki, Takayasu's,

5. Metabolic - Renal failure, Alport's, Renal transplantation, Renal Tubular Acidosis, DM, IgA nephropathy, Hyperlipidemia, Hypothyroidism, Refsum's

6. Miscellaneous - ulcerative colitis, Sarcoidosis, Scleroderma

7. Neoplastic

8. Skeletal system & Otic capsule

   1. Secondary deposit from breast & prostate, multiple myeloma

   2. Osteoma of IAC

9. Ototoxicity – (ABCDEFGHI-KLMNOP QRSTUV)

   A- Antibiotic – Aminoglycoside, vancomycin, viomycin, minocycline,

   B- Bromocriptine, Beta blockers, Barbiturates, Bumetanide

   C- Cytotoxic drugs, carbon monoxide intoxication (U shaped audiogram) Cisplatin

   D- Dantrolene

   E- Erythromycin, Ethacrynic acid

   F- Furosemide

   G- Gentamicin - vestibular toxic

   H- Heparin (Anti heparin drugs) Hexadimethrine bromide

   I- Interferon alpha & Beta

   K- Kanamycin - cochlear toxic

   L- Loop diuretics

   M- Mianerin, Marichuana

   N- Nicotine

   O- Oral contraceptives pill - Injection depo progesterone

   P- Phenytoin, practolol

   Q- Quinine

R- revaccination for smallpox, Rabies Injection

S- Salicylates - Flattish Curve

T- Tobacco and TB drugs (Streptomycin), Tobramycin, Topical drugs

V- Vaccination - Tetanus Antitoxin, whooping cough vaccination

10. Hematological

1) iron deficiency Anemia, Megaloblastic, Fanconi's, Pernicious, Aplastic Anemia

2) Polycythemia vera, thalassemia, Sickle cell

3) Waldenstrom's Macroglobulinemia

4) Leukemia – ALL

5) Cryoglobulinemia

COMMON PATHOLOGY IN SNHL

1. Acute Labyrinthitis

2. endoLymphatic Hydrops

3. Focal proliferative Of Fibrous tissue & Bone

4. Diffuse proliferative Of Fibrous tissue & Bone

5. Retrogradeneurodegeneration

GENETIC CAUSES OF CONDUCTIVE DEAFNESS (ADAPT ON HCG-MD)

1. Apert's syndrome & Achondroplasia

2. Down's Syndrome

3. Pierre - Robin Syndrome (Hypoplasia Mandible, cleft palate, glossoptosis)

4. Treacher-Collins syndrome

5. Osteogenesis Imperfecta

6. Nager syndrome

   7. Hemifacial microsomia

   8. Crouzon syndrome (parrot - beak nose)

   9. Goldenhars syndrome (epibulbar Dermoid)

   10. Marfan's Duane syndrome

2. CONGENITAL ABNORMALITIES CHL - (5 I'S)

1. Idiopathic - Aberrant Facial nerve, persistent stapedial artery congenital absence of OW and RW

2. Inheritance - Otosclerosis

3. Infection (prenatal)- Rubella & Congenital syphilis

4. Iatrogenic - Alcohol, Phenytoin and Vit A derivative

5. Ingestion - intra amniotic fluid aspiration

3. CONGENITAL CAUSES OF CHL

1. Minor external & Middle ear malformation (group I)

2. Moderate external & middle ear malformation - microtia (Type I II III)

3. Severe external & Middle ear malformation

4. EAC atresia UL/BL, partial or complete, Osseous or membranous

5. Ossicular malformation - Cong M-I fixation & Malleus abnormality

4. CAUSES OF ACQUIRED CONDUCTIVE DEAFNESS

1. EAC causes -1. Wax & keratosis obturans

   2. Impacted FB

3. Otitis Externa & Malignant otitis externa

4. Tumor – Benign, Malignant

5. Canal Atresia

2. Tympanic Membrane -

1. Bullous myringitis

2. Myringosclerosis

3. Granular Myringitis

4. Traumatic rupture of tm

5. Perforation of tm

3. Middle ear causes -

1. ASOM, CSOM, OME, Acute necrotizing otitis media and Adhesive otitis media

2. Trauma – Hemotympanum, Barotrauma

3. Ossicular dislocation

4. Otosclerosis & Tympanosclerosis

5. Growth – Aural polyp, Glomus & Cancer

4. ET & Nasopharynx causes -

1. Tubal catarrh

2. ET dysfunction

3. Barotrauma

4. Adenoids

5. Growth in Nasopharynx – NPC

5. Metabolic & systemic causes-

1. Wegener's granulomatosis

2. Relapsing polychondritis

3. Fibrous dysplasia

4. Eosinophilic granuloma

5. Sarcoidosis

5. MISCELLANEOUS CAUSES OF CHL – (5 C' S)

1. Congenital cholesteatoma

2. cilia syndrome

3. Cystic Fibrosis

4. Cleft palate

5. Carcinoma- rhabdomyosarcoma & fibrous dysplasia

CLINICAL FEATURES OF TREACHER – COLLINS SYNDROME

(1) Face-   1. Hypoplasia of malar borne

2. Hypoplasia of mandible

3. Shrunken cheek

4. Fish mouth

5. Nose is normal but prominent

(2) Eye   1. Sloping supraorbital ridge

2. Microphthalmia

3. Coloboma

4. Antimongoloid slant of palpebral fissure

(3) External Ear

- Accessory tubercles, Microtia & Atresia EAC

(4) Middle Ear

- ossicular discontinuity, CHL, TM replace by bony plate

(5) Inner Ear - Normal

JAHRSDOERFER GRADING (SELECTION OF PTS FOR SURGICAL CORRECTION IN CHL)

1. Presence of stapes 2
2. Open OW   1
3. Middle Ear space   1
4. Facial nerves   1
5. M-I complex   1
6. mastoid air cell   1
7. I-S connection   1
8. RW   1
9. Auricular appendages 1

TOTAL SCORE   10

    (SCORE <5 -NO

    SCORE >7-YES

REFERRED OTALGIA

[GATE theory- the wider spread diffuse monosynaptic input to the cells of the substantia gelatinosa of the spinal cord, often from relatively distant afferents, and it is suggested that this diffuse input is normally inhibited by presynaptic gate mechanisms, but may be triggered if stimulus is sufficiently intense.]

1. Tonsillitis, parotitis, mumps
2. Nasal polyps, sinusitis, thyroid disease
3. Tuberculosis of the larynx, teeth, oral ulcer, TM joint
4. Elongated Styloid process
5. Myocardial ischemia, malignancy of pyriform fossa

16

NOISE INDUCED HEARING LOSS

1. Boiler's deafness, Black-Simth deafness & immersion blast

2. Classification a) Noise induced temporary threshold shift (24-36 hrs)

    b) Noise induced permanent threshold shift

    c) Acute Acoustic trauma

3. PTA

    -Auditory notch at 4 KHZ in case of SNHL

    -Auditory notch at 2 KHZ in immersion blast

    -Abrupt slope

    -Symmetrical High frequency Hearing loss

4. Structural changes are basilar membrane fixed, degeneration of outer hair cell softening of cuticular plate of hair cells and Stereocilia damaged.

5. Hydropic Ear, symphonic, musicians, violinists and pt on Aspirin, more risky individuals for noise induced HL

"Inner hair cells are more resistant to acoustic trauma,"

17
PRESBYCUSIS

1. Neural   - Degeneration & loss of neural elements

                     - Mechanical

                     - degeneration or inefficiency of inner ear supporting elements

2. Sensory   - Degeneration & loss of hair cells

                     - Metabolic -Inner ear biochemical defect

3. Mixed   - Intermediate presbycusis

4. Atrophy of stria vascularis

                     - flat Audiogram

5. Inner Ear Conductive deafness

                     -Ski-slope audiogram

TREATMENT FOR SUDDEN SNHL

1. Oral prednisolone and oral Nicotinic acid and pentoxifylline

2. Low molecular weight Dextran and Multivitamins infusion

3. Carbogen (5% co2 + 95% Oxygen)

4. Hyperbaric Oxygen

5. Stellate Ganglion block.

18

COCHLEAR IMPLANTS

THE BASIC PARTS OF COCHLEAR IMPLANTS (MASTRE)

1. Microphone
2. Speech processor

    Single Channel - House, MED-EL

    Multiple Channel (LIMCA), Laura, Ineraid, MXM

    Clarion, Nucleus
3. Transmitter coil – Transcutaneous device
4. Receiver coil – implanted into the bone of the skull behind the ear
5. Electrodes (4-22)

    - Extracochlear - Round window, basal turn of cochlea

    - Intra cochlear- (Scala Tympani)

    - Monopolar and Bipolar

INDICATION OF COCHLEAR IMPLANTS

1. Congenital deaf children
2. Acquired pre lingually deaf children – Meningitis labyrinthitis ossificans
3. Acquired post lingually deaf children – 6 to 12 year age
4. Acquired pre lingually deaf adults
5. Acquired post lingually deaf adults -> 12 year

SURGICAL STEPS IN COCHLEAR IMPLANT

1. Post auricular Incision Under General Anaesthesia
2. Complete mastoidectomy and A Seat for the inner coil is created in the region of sinodural angle
3. Facial recess is exposed.
4. The overhang of round window niche is removed
5. 0.7 mm to 0.8 mm fenestra created Anteroinferiorly to Round window

COCHLEAR IMPLANT TEAM

1. Surgeons
2. Audiological Scientists & Speech, Language therapists
3. Teachers of the deaf
4. Medical physicists
5. Administrator

CHILDREN'S COCHLEAR IMPLANT PROFILE (CHIP)

Factors to select the Patient

1. Chronological age, duration of deafness
2. Medical radiological findings, functional hearing level
3. Multiple handicapping condition, availability services
4. Speech – language abilities, family structure & support
5. Parent – child expectations, Education environment & cognitive hearing style

"A minimum of a six months trial with appropriate amplification and rehabilitation before surgery "

CT-TEMPORAL BONE (THIN-SECTION HRCT) IN IMPLANTS

1. The thickness of the parietal bone
2. The degree of pneumatization of the mastoid
3. Measurement of size of the facial recess
4. Description of the size and orientation of the round window niche
5. The patency of the basal turn of Cochlea

SPECIAL ASPECTS OF COCHLEAR IMPLANT CHILDREN

1. Skull growth maximum at 2 years of age
2. Acute otitis media risk of spread of infection
3. Long-term effects of electrical stimulation – need not adversely affect the residual auditory nerve fibers
4. Longevity of the implanted device – reimplantation
5. Implant device failure

SURGICAL IMPORTANT POINTS IN COCHLEAR IMPLANTS

1. Duration of surgery 3-4 hrs, Hospital stay 3-4 days
2. Not to raise a separate periosteal flap (Nottingham)
3. The cochleostomy is sealed with small piece of muscle
4. Wounds are irrigated with a tetracycline solution. Subcuticular sutures to close wounds. A firm head dressing is applied for 48 hours in order to reduce the risk of Hematoma formation and drains are not used
5. Reverse Stenvers view X-ray to demonstrate the position of the electrode after surgery

COMPLICATION OF COCHLEAR IMPLANT SURGERY

1. Facial palsies
2. Flap Necrosis
3. Failure device
4. Cholesteatoma
5. Total ossification

MAP (MEMORY ACCESS PROCESSOR) IN REHABILITATION OF POST -OP COCHLEAR IMPLANT SURGERY

- Switch on & tuning after one month of surgery

1. Disengaged – The child's visual attention is not on the speaker but on other activities
2. Engaged – The child starts to look at the speaker or at the object of discourse
3. Structured looking – The child now starts to look at the speaker and takes his 'Turn' in conversation
4. Structured vocalization – Vocalizations become more word like and are more likely to take place in turns
5. Equal conversational partnership – The child now demonstrates initiative and autonomy in the conversation

COMMUNICATION METHODS IN DEAF CHILDREN

1. Auralism & oralism
2. Finger spelling
3. Cued speech

4. Signing systems (Manualism) – British sign language, Signed English Paget – Gorman sign system & Maketon

5. Total communication

ABI (AUDITORY BRAINSTEM IMPLANT) HOUSE & HISTELBERG'S 1979

1. It is surgically implanted central neural auditory prosthesis

2. Indication
    a) NF type 2
    b) After Schwannoma surgery
    c) Bilateral Cochlear nerves Avulsion by trauma
    d) Complete ossification of cochlea
    e) Severe cochlear malformation

3. The External components are microphone, battery, speech processor, external magnet & Transmitter antenna. -The internal components are internal magnet, Antenna, receiver – Stimulator and an electrode array

4. It is kept is the lateral recess of the fourth ventricle near dorsal cochlear Nucleus

5. Translabyrinth or retro sigmoid approach

BAHA

1. Bone anchored hearing aid is a combination of a Brainmark titanium implant and a bone conduction hearing aid.

2. Indicated in congenital aural atresia and a severe conductive hearing loss

3. Parts are
    1. Volume & tone control
    2. Microphone & piston

3. Security coupling with O-ring

4. Connection Screw & cover screw

5. Titanium coupling & fixture

4. Advantages are

1. Patient satisfaction is very high because of quality of sound

2. Binaural nature

3. Comfort

4. Cosmetic advantage of the aid which can be concealed in the hair

5. If acts not only for conductive hearing loss but will help in sensorineural hearing loss also

5. Vibratory energy reaching the cochlea causes alternate compression and expansion of the cochlear shell

"This aid wearing time more than 12 hours/day"

19
OTOSCLEROSIS

ETIOLOGY OF OTOSCLEROSIS

1. (VITAMEH)

    Vascular

    immune disorders

    infection

    Trauma

    Anatomical

    Metabolic

    Embryology

    HPE

2. Unstable rests of Embryonic cartilage with in labyrinth capsule & Fissure [↑Antitype II collagen Ab)

3. More common in women than men 2:1,

    unilateral otosclerosis common in men

    Bilateral otosclerosis common in women

4. Measles Virus

5. Autosomal dominant with incomplete penetrance

    6p 7q 15q, more common in Caucasian races.

SITE OF OTOSCLEROSIS

1) OW – 85% & RW – 50%

2) Fossula Anti fenestrum - Cozzolino's zone

3) Processus Cochleariformis

4) Bulge of the Promontory

5) Fossula post fenestram, base of styloid process, petrosquamous suture, SSC and inter cochlear

TYPE OF OTOSCLEROSIS

1) Rim fixed anteriorly - center Free

2) Biscuits or rice-grain- footplate with delineated margins

3) Solid foot plate- partly or spuriously

4) Obliterative – totally obscures foot plate

5) Malignant otosclerosis –oval window, round window & cochlear body

ENZYMES IN OTOSCLEROTIC FOCI

1. Alpha- Chymotrypsin & Trypsin

2. Phosphatase

3. Collagenase & Cathepsin D

4. Lactic Dehydrogenase

5. Ribonuclease

GROSS APPEARANCE OF FOOT PLATE

Type O   - Normal

Type I   - Minimally fixed & can be moved

Type II   - Footplate thin – Milky opalescence

Type III   - Foot plate thick- chalky and opaque

Type IV   - Foot plate very thick- fixed

CLINICAL FEATURES OF OTOSCLEROSIS

1.	Deafness	-	Conductive Hearing loss >25-30 dB
2.	Paracusis Willisii	-	Hearing better in noisy Surroundings as they raise their voices above the noise level
3.	Voice	-	Quiet & Good tone – monotonous voice because they hear their own voice by bone conduction
4.	Tinnitus	-	More common in early stage or commonly seen in SN degeneration -roaring, hissing or pulsatile type
5.	Vertigo	-	Action of toxic enzyme, BPPV, vestibular hydrops or involvement of the vestibular aqueduct

SIGNS OF OTOSCLEROSIS

1. TM – Normal, mint condition, Atrophic, thickened rigid or immobile

2. Prominent blood vessels seen in sub mucosal layer of mucous membrane of the promontory (Schwartz sign)

3. Rinne negative, weber -lateralized to the affected ear, ABC not reduced, Gelle & Bing test positive

4. Carhart's Notch - Bone conduction threshold at 2 KHZ, it reflects a loss in the inertial component of the stapes footplate

5. Impedance Audiometry – As type of Tympanogram with absent stapedial reflex static compliance- less than 0.2 cm² – thick foot plate - more than 0.6 cm²- thin foot plate "

SHAMBAUGH DIAGNOSIS OF SNHL IN OTOSCLEROSIS

1. A positive Schwartze sign in one or both ears

2. A family H/o surgically confirmed stapedial otosclerosis

3. The presence of symmetrical SNHL with presence of stapes fixation one side of ear

4. A flat, rising or cookie – bite Audiogram with good speech discrimination

5. Pure SNHL begins insidiously in early, or middle, adult life and progresses with no apparent cause.

OTOSCLEROSIS INNER EAR SYNDROME

1) Episodic vertigo 20 Mins to 6 Hours

2) Absence of nystagmus

3) Normal caloric response

4) No positional vertigo

5) PTA-Conductive hearing loss, normal speech & Absence of recruitment

DIFFERENTIAL DIAGNOSIS OF OTOSCLEROSIS (CSOM-PT)

1) Congenital Cholesteatoma, Congenital foot plate fixation CSF-Hyrtl'S Fistula (Tympano Meningeal duct)

2) Secretory otitis media, **S**clerosis (**T**ympanosclerosis & **M**yringosclerosis)

3) **O**ssicular discontinuity, **O**steogenesis Imperfecta

4) **M**alleus incus fixed, **m**iddle **E**ar fibrosis [Adhesions]

5) **P**aget's Disease, **P**ersistent Stapedial artery

CAUSES OF SNHL IN OTOSCLEROSIS

1. Bony Invasion of the scala tympani

2. Ruedi Theory (ottomayer's) Vascularis shunts between otosclerotic blood vessels & Spiral capillaries (Circulatory changes)

3. Nager's theory -Stimulation of the osteoblastic activity of the endosteal capsule

4. Damage to the cochlea by toxic metabolites from the abnormal bone via canaliculi

5. Enzymatic concept – Proteases or Hydrolases enter the labyrinthine fluids

INDICATION FOR Na F IN OTOSCLEROSIS

1. patients with surgically confirmed otosclerosis who show progressive SNHL disproportionate to age

2. Cochlear Otosclerosis

3. Radiological Demonstration of spongiotic changes (double ring) in the cochlear capsule

4. Patients with a positive Schwartze sign

5. Malignant otosclerosis

CONTRA INDICATION OF Na F

1. Renal failure
2. Chronic rheumatoid Arthritis
3. Child, Pregnant or Lactating mother
4. Allergy
5. Skeletal fluorosis

Na F (SODIUM FLUORIDE) THERAPY

1. NaF 50 mg for 2 years
2. ↓ Osteoclastic (bone resorption) and
3. ↑ Osteoblastic (Bone formation)
4. Supplemented with calcium and Vit D
5. Promotes recalcification and reduce bone remodeling
6. Adverse effects – Gastric disturbance, Increase of joint symptoms, chronic arthritis and skeletal fluorosis

TREATMENT OF OTOSCLEROSIS

1. Medical – NaF
2. Hearing aids
3. Osseous implanted hearing aids
4. Stapedectomy or Stapedotomy (First stapedectomy done by Jack of Boston and Modern stapedotomy done by John Shea 1958.
5. Fenestration operation done previously by Jenkins& Lempert

INDICATION OF STAPEDOTOMY

1. Bone conduction   0-25 dB

| 2. | Air conduction | 45-65 dB |
| 3. | Air – Bone Gap at least | 15 dB |

4. Speech Discrimination score more than 60%

5. Clinical otosclerosis

CONTRAINDICATION OF STAPEDECTOMY

1. Child, old age, pregnancy, Infection (Otitis externa, Chronic Otitis Media)

2. General Medical condition – Diabetic Mellitus, Bleeding Disorder & Unfit for surgery

3. Tympanosclerosis causing stapes fixation

4. unilateral otosclerosis, only hearing Ear, Second Ear stapedectomy or poor Air-Bone gap

5. labyrinthine Hydrops & positive Schwartze sign

OPERATIVE COUNSELING FOR STAPEDECTOMY

1. Good hearing improvement 85%, slight improvement 15%, SNHL 5% and Dead ear

2. Slight vertigo for a few days after surgery

3. Transient weakness of facial muscles

4. Alteration of taste

5. Avoid Noise, flying for at least 2 weeks, strenuous exercise and lifting of heavy weights

STEPS OF STAPEDECTOMY PROCEDURE

1. Triangular Tympanomeatal flap raised, Chorda tympani nerve is freed from mucosal attachment.

2. Posterior bony overhang removed till pyramid base seen

3. The stapes head separated from the lenticular process after dividing stapes tendon

4. Stapes crura removed from Footplate and 2 mm strip of mucosa around oval window is removed

5. Foot plate transected transversely and the prosthesis placed between long process of incus and Oval Window, the defect closed by vein or Ear lobe fat graft.

MODIFIED STAPES SURGERY

1. Stapedotomy - Defect is created on posterior half of footplate [because Acoustic gain is more through posterior half) about 1 mm larger in its diameter than that of the preferred prosthesis, only 0.25 mm tip entered into peri lymphatic space.

   (male-5 mm length 0.5 mm diameter, female-4.5 mm & 0.4 mm) "The length of prosthesis measured from under surface of long process of incus to upper surface of the footplate "

2. Revised stapedotomy –

3. Laser stapedotomy – Perkins 1980

4. Preserve the stapes tendon with posterior crura to prevents the hyperacusis

5. STAMP - Laser Stapedotomy minus prosthesis, opening is sealed with ear lobe fat

PROBLEMS FOUND AT STAPES OPERATION

1. Abnormal Facial nerve and persistent stapedial artery

2. Perilymph flooding (Gusher) & floating or submerged foot plate

3. Damage to chorda & Tympanic membrane

4. Obliterative otosclerosis & Narrowed Oval window niche

5. Presence of blood in the vestibule

CAUSES OF PERSISTENT POST OP CONDUCTIVE HL

1. Loosely articulated prosthesis

2. Incus necrosis

3. Disarticulated prosthesis

4. Medially displaced prosthesis

5. Prosthesis length is inadequate

CAUSES OF IMMEDIATE SNHL AFTER STAPES SURGERY

1. Acoustic trauma from drilling

2. Excessive movement of the stapes producing a hydraulic effect

3. Rupture of the membranous inner Ear

4. Rapid loss of perilymph & floating foot plate

5. Presence of blood or bone dust in the vestibule

CAUSES OF DELAYED SNHL AFTER STAPES SURGERY

1. Energy transmission to the cochlea

2. Effects of the sensory apparatus

3. Loss of outer hair cell & First order neurons

4. Noise Exposure leads to distortion of hair cells, Degenerative changes & reduction of ribonucleic acid

5. Mechanical aspects – the sudden loss of peri lymphatic pressure affect ionic transport and microcirculation by histamine release

COMPLICATION OF STAPES SURGERY

1. Conductive hearing loss
2. Immediate severe SNHL, Delayed SNHL & Chronic progressive SNHL
3. Perilymph Fistula & Bell's Palsy
4. TM Perforation & injury to Chorda tympani nerve
5. Reparative granuloma

TYPES OF STAPES PROSTHESIS

1. Teflon -Prosthesis length in measured from under surface of the long process of incus to upper surface of foot plate + 0.5 mm. (0.5 mm depth is safety in the vestibule) Maximum acoustic gain noted if fenestration is made in posterior half of the foot plate
2. Schuknecht prosthesis - fat & wire prosthesis is best for pilots
3. Stainless steel – Titanium
4. Lippy moon Robison prosthesis – Malleus to foot plate
5. Lensiki prosthesis –– Malleus to foot plate

STAPES

1. Weight - 2.86 mg
2. Length of Stapes - 2.64 mm-3.37 mm
3. Height of stapes - (3.2 mm) Height of Footplate – (1.4 mm)

4. Width of stapes - (1.41 mm) Width of foot plate – (1.9 mm)

5. Thickness of foot plate - 0.4 mm

20

MENIERE'S DISEASE

TYPES OF MENIERE'S DISEASE

1. Meniere's Disease – Certain, Definite, Probable & Possible

2. Atypical Meniere's Disease

3. Cochlear Meniere's & Vestibular Meniere's

4. Lermoyez Syndrome – Sudden SNHL Improve after vertigo

5. Tumarkin's otolithic catastrophe or Drop attack

   Sudden unexplained fall without loss a consciousness or vertigo

   Meyerhott's type – Abnormal oculovestibular response

SYMPTOMS OF MENIERE'S DISEASE

1. Vertigo (Episodic) -20 Minutes to 24 hours -Horizontal

   Nystagmus

   -Associated with nausea & Vomiting

2. Hearing loss -SNHL, fluctuating Hearing loss, Progressive SNHL, low frequency & High frequency Hearing loss (Tent or Peaked PTA) (Inverted V shape)

3. Tinnitus   - Continuous not pulsatile

4. Aural fullness

5. Diplacusis & Dysacusis.

SHEA FIRE STAGE OF MENIERE'S DISEASE

Stage I   -   Solely cochlear symptom

Stage II   -   Progressively Cochlear Symptoms

Stage III   -   Vestibular symptoms

Stage VI   -   Both Cochlear & vestibular symptoms

Stage V   -   End Stage Meniere's disease

PATHOPHYSIOLOGY OF MENIERE'S DISEASE

1. Prodromal stage of Endolymphatic Sac Distention

2. Leading to thin and Atrophy of Reissner's membrane and saccular wall

3. Rupture of Membrane release endolymph and exposed to K^+ rich endolymph on sensory neural structure

4. Sudden hearing loss & Vertigo

5. Peri lymphatic compartment returns to normal, rupture heals, all symptoms disappear.

CAUSES OF PRIMARY MENIERE'S DESERVE

1. Genetic & Anatomical -HLA-DP2 6P

   -Autosomal Dominant

   -small vestibular aqueduct

2. Traumatic – Biochemical dysfunction of cells and debris in to Endolymphatic duct Causing obstruction

3. Viral infection – HSV I & Enterovirus

4. Allergy & Autoimmunity

5. Psychosomatic and personality Features

CAUSES OF SECONDARY ENDOLYMPHATIC HYDROPS

1. Developmental insult – Embryopathy, Mondini dysplasia

2. Abnormal metabolic, endocrine and fluid balance, decrease and increase in glycemia, decrease in potassium, increase in lipoprotein, decrease in thyroid, and hemodialysis.

3. Viral and autoimmunity- Cogans, Measles, Mumps

4. Otosclerosis and chronic otitis media

5. Syphilis, Leukemia, Shy-Drager syndrome, Temporal arteritis

DIFFERENTIAL DIAGNOSIS OF MENIERE'S DISEASE- PERIPHERAL CAUSES

1. BPPV

2. Vestibular Neuronitis

3. Labyrinthitis

4. Perilymph Fistula

5. Otosclerosis & Migraine

TEST FOR MENIERE'S DISEASE

1. PTA - Inverted 'V' Shape Audiogram

   Type-II Bekesy Audiometry.

2. Caloric test-canal paresis or preponderance

3. Glycerol test – 60 ml of 95% Glycerol oral Intake with lime juice then Serial PTA taken with a gap of one hour

4. OAE and BERA – Absent cochlear Echo & Vth wave always present, interpeak Latency is less than 1 m sec, early wave absent. Increased traveling wave velocity

5. Electrocochleography

   1. Cochlear Microphonic is lower

   2. AP threshold is variable

   3. Summation potential tends to be increased

   4. SP/AP ratio is more than 0.5

   5. SP Amplitude More than 3 mv

LABYRINTHINE SEDATIVE

1. Antihistamines - Cinnarazine, Promethazine, Meclizine

2. Phenothiazines - Prochlorperazine

3. Benzodiazepines - Diazepam, Lorazepam & Amitriptyline

4. Scopolamines - Transdermal Sublingual

5. Antidopaminergic - Droperidol

DRUGS USED FOR MENIERE'S DISEASE (INCREASE MICROCIRCULATION)

1. Betahistine 24 mg bd

2. ATP, Amyl nitrate, Isosorbide & Nitroglycerine

3. Nicotinamide, Dipyradamole, Papaverine

4. Carbogen & Flunarizine

5. Steroids & Diuretics

SURGICAL TREATMENT FOR MENIERE'S DISEASE

1. Procedures involving hearing preservation and vestibular preservation

   1. a) Portmann's operation – Endolymphatic Sac decompression by opening the sac

b) Naito creating an Endolymphatic – subarachnoid fistula

c) Shambaugh Decompression without opening sac

d) Shea used Teflon film

e) Avenberg used silastic sheet

Fick and Cody Tack procedures designed to create a fistula in saccule via oval window

2. Procedures involving hearing preservation and vestibular ablation

    1. Sectioning the 8th CN

    2. Vestibular Nerve Section via middle fossa, Retro sigmoid and retro labyrinthine approach.

    3. Singular neurectomy (Gacek's)

    4. Cochleo Sacculotomy

    5. Stapedectomy- Sacculotomy

3. Procedures involving chemical ablation of the vestibular end organ

    1. Intra tympanic streptomycin (Schuknecht)

    2. Intra tympanic Gentamicin (Beck) 0.8 ml (out of 26.4 mg/ ml) into middle Ear)

4. Procedures involving hearing & Vestibular ablation of the vestibular End organ

    1. Ultrasonic irradiation to labyrinth

    2. Cryosurgery (Wolfson)

5. Procedures involving hearing & Vestibular ablation

    1. Trans tympanic Labyrinthectomy

    2. Trans canal Labyrinthectomy

    3. Trans meatal Labyrinthectomy

4. Trans mastoid Labyrinthectomy

5. Trans labyrinthine vestibular neurectomy

ENDOLYMPHATIC SAC SURGICAL ANATOMY

1. Pear shape white in color (Dura is gray) double layer dura

2. Donaldson's line – imaginary line bisecting the posterior semicircular canal up to sigmoid sinus

3. Sac related posterior by sinus,

   Inferiorly by Jugular,

   Anteriorly by retro facial,

   Superiorly by SCC

4. Location depends on amount of periaqueductal pneumatization

5. ES is Glistening Smooth moist structure

21

GLOMUS TUMORS

FEATURES OF GLOMUS TUMORS

-Glomus Tympanicus

-Glomus Jugulare

1. Highly Vascular, slow growing tumor

2. Well – Defined thin fibrous capsule

3. Locally invasive & destructive of Fallopian canal

4. Glomus cells are derivatives of non-chromatin ganglionic of neuroectodermal origin & have secretory capacity (VMA) as well.

5. More common in female & multi centricity

SITE OF GLOMUS CELL BODIES

1. Adventitia of the Jugular bulb

2. Promontory

3. Tympani branch of the IX CN

4. Auricular Branch of the X CN

5. It is Supplied by non-Medullated Sensory Fibers and Ascending pharyngeal artery

SYMPTOMS OF GLOMUS TUMORS

1. Pulsatile objective tinnitus

2. Conductive deafness

3. Rising Sun sign behind the TM- Red mass

4. Brown's Sign – Blanching of tumor mass with pneumatic otoscopy

5. Vertigo and CN palsies, bleeding from Ear & Otologic headache

CLASSIFICATION OF GLOMUS TUMORS

1. Lundgren -Glomus Jugulare - Glomus tympanicus

2. Alford & Guilford

3. Oldring & Fisch

4. Fisch & Mattox

5. Jackson & Glasscock

OLDRING & FISCH CLASSIFICATION

1. Type A - localized to middle Ear

2. Type B- Tympanomastoid tumor with no destruction to bone in Infralabyrinthine part

3. Type C- Tumor with destruction of bone in infra labyrinthine part

4. Type D1 - Intracranial extension less than 2 cm

5. Type D2 - Intracranial Extension more than 2 Cm.

SPREAD OF GLOMUS TUMOR

1. Anteriorly - Nasopharynx via ET

2. Medially - Labyrinth & IAC

3. Superiorly - Intracranial via hypotympanum & protympanum

4. Laterally - EAC via TM Perforation

5. Inferiorly - IJV & Sigmoid sinus, carotid

INVESTIGATION OF GLOMUS TUMORS

1. X-ray mastoid – Jagged erosion of Jugular bulb with mastoid sclerosis

2. CT- Phelp's Sign – Absence of crotch bone between carotid canal &   Jugular fossa

3. CT- Moth -eaten appearance of bony rim

4. MRI – Salt & Pepper appearance (mixed hypo tense & iso tense on T1)

5. MRA, arteriography Retrograde, venography, PTA.

TREATMENT FOR GLOMUS TUMOR

1. No Active treatment & Continuous observation

2. Primary Radiotherapy 4000-5000 cGy over a 3-4 week

3. Transmeatal Approach – type A tumor

4. Extended facial recess approach – type B tumor

5. Infra Temporal fossa & posterolateral approach with upper cervical incision Posterior craniotomy -Type C & Type D tumor

BASIC STEPS OF FISCH INFRATEMPORAL FOSSA APPROACH

1. Post aural incision is extended superiorly & inferiorly into the neck.

2. Cartilaginous meatus is transected and closed off as a blind – Ending Sac with mobilization of the peripheral branches of facial nerve with Anterior transposition of facial nerve

3. Control ligatures are placed around the ICA, IJV, lower cranial nerves

4. Subtotal petrosectomy done with packing off the sigmoid sinus, if possible medial wall of the sinus is preserved.

5. Dural defect is repaired with facia & ET closed with bone wax and whole cavity filled with a free fat graft

22
VERTIGO

CLASSIFICATION OF DIZZINESS

1. Single episode with or without cochlear symptoms and without cochlear symptom with or without associate symptoms,

2. recurrent attack with or without cochlear symptoms & without cochlear symptoms with or without associate symptoms

3. recurrent attack with cochlear symptoms with or without associated symptoms

4. Continue imbalance with or without cochlear symptoms & without cochlear symptom with or without associated symptoms

5. Continue imbalance with cochlear symptoms with or without associated symptoms

ETIOLOGY OF VERTIGO

(ONE VIP iS The HM)

1. Otological
    1. Acoustic Neuroma, vestibular neuritis
    2. Benign Paroxysmal Positional vertigo
    3. Cholesteatoma, Middle ear disease, labyrinthitis
    4. Tuberculosis, Temporal lobe lesions, syphilis, glomus

5. Meniere's Otosclerosis, Ramsay Hunt syndrome

2. Neurological 1. Cerebellopontine angle, pontine, thalamic medullary, cerebellar, cerebral & internal capsule lesions

2. Epilepsy, Parkinsonism, multiple sclerosis

3. Subdural & Extradural hematoma, injury

4. Hydrocephalus, meningitis, Borellia

5. Shy Drager & Stede – Richandson syndrome

3. Endocrine -> Hypothyroidism & Hypoglycemia

4. Vascular ->
1. Wallenberg's and vertebrobasilar insufficiency

2. Subclavian steal syndrome & Vasculitis

3. Syncope & postural Hypotension

4. Carotid sinus syndrome and cardiac dysrhythmia

5. Mechanical cardiac dysfunction

Visual -> Ocular & Retro orbital pathology & Diplopia

5. Iatrogenic -> Drugs induce hypotension, confusion, central vestibular lesions, Inappropriate of lens, cervical collar & walking aids

6. Psychogenic

7. Skeletal   - Osteoarthritis, Paget's cervical abnormalities

8. Toxin   - Ethanol, carbon monoxide

9. Hematological - Anemia, hemoglobinopathies, Hyper-
viscosity

10. Metastatic from nasopharynx ear

Classification of vertigo

1. Short-lived (Seconds) Episodic rotatory vertigo

   - Stimulation or depression of labyrinth (ABCPVL)

   a. BPPV

   b. Labyrinthine fistula

   c. Caloric Effect & **A**lternobaric vertigo

   d. Post – concussion syndrome & Vestibulobasilar
   insufficiency

   e. Cervical vertigo & Coriolis phenomenon (Stimulation
   of another pair of semicircular canal while First pair
   is still being stimulated)

2. Hours episodic rotatory vertigo (Minutes to 24 hours)

   – Metabolic failure (MSD)

   a. Meniere's disease

   b. Syphilitic Labyrinthitis

   c. Delayed endolymphatic hydrops

   d. Decompensation of previous vestibular lesion

   e. following middle ear surgery

3. Prolonged (weeks) rotatory vertigo

   – Destructive lesions

   a. Vestibular neuronitis

b. Labyrinthitis

c. Vascular lesion

d. Metastatic deposits in Cerebellopontine angle

e. Trauma by head injury, Ear surgery, vestibular neurectomy and labyrinthectomy

4. Short-lived episodic unsteadiness

   – Physiological overload

   a. Rapid movement

   b. Abnormal input – visual

   c. Visual inadequacies

   d. Vestibular inadequacies

   e. Proprioceptive inadequacies

5. Hours Episodic unsteadiness

   – Temporary impairment of central connection

   a. Drugs – self- inflicted or Iatrogenic

   b. Travel sickness

   c. Peri lymphatic Fistula & CSOM active stage

   d. De-compensation of Pre-Existing lesion

   e. Hyperventilation & Functional

6. Prolonged unsteadiness

   a. The Elderly

   b. CNS tumor – Schwannoma

   c. Floating females

   d. Toxic products from chronic otitis media

   e. Drugs – Anticonvulsants

   – Gentamicin

VERTIGO FOLLOWING HEAD INJURY

1. Post – Concussion Syndrome
2. BPPV & Perilymph Fistula
3. Destructive labyrinthine lesions
4. Delayed hydrops
5. Functional

INVESTIGATION FOR VERTIGO

1. PTA & Speech discrimination score
2. Electronystagmography
3. Caloric tests & Butterfly chart
4. Radiological – CT MRI

Dynamic Posturography & Video Head impulse test (VHIT)

TREATMENT OF VERTIGO

1. Treat or eliminate the cause
2. Suppress the vestibular system with drugs
3. Suppress the patient Emotional Reaction and Acceptance of the problem
4. Wait for compensation or eliminate the offending labyrinth
5. Surgery

    a. Meniere's – Sac decompression

    b. Labyrinthine Fistula – Closed with Grafts

    c. Labyrinthectomy

    d. Vestibular nerve section – BPPV

    e. -> Gacek Procedure – section of the

    (Singular nerve) Posterior ampullary nerve

-> Parnes & Mc Clure procedure – Approach to posterior SCC – 2 mm fenestration leaving membranous labyrinth & closed with bone paste

BENIGN PAROXYSMAL POSITIONAL VERTIGO

Features of BPPV

1. Latent period is Few Seconds

2. Distress present

3. On sitting up again similar events with nystagmus in opposite direction

4. Fatigability – Nystagmus & dizziness stop with fatigability testing

5. direction of nystagmus is rotatory and Anticlockwise with Right Ear down & clockwise with Ear down (Horizontal) Duration of nystagmus less than 30 seconds

BENIGN PAROXYSMAL POSITIONAL VERTIGO

1. Cupulolithiasis - More common in female

2. Etiology - Idiopathic, Degenerative, Trauma viral, Secondary to Meniere & Labyrinthitis After Ear supply & after prolonged bed rest

3. Calcium carbonate crystals from saccula or utricular otoconia impinge on the cupula of the posterior semi-circular canal (Most dependent canal)

4. Diagnosis by Dix- Hallpike maneuver

5. Treated by Epley's maneuver

   - Canalith repositioning Procedure (CRP)

   "Presbyastasis – The disequilibrium of aging"

STEPS IN EPLEY'S MANEUVER

Example; Left ear

1. The patient is seated with head erect and facing forwards (otolith debris lie freely in posterior semicircular canal)

2. The head is turned 45° to the left and Patient is brought to the supine position such that head remains extended beyond the Edge of the table at 45° to horizontal (otolith debris towards center of Posterior Semicircular canal)

3. The head is tuned 90° to right side (otolith debris reaches the common crus)

4. The head and body are rotated to right side until the body is turned to 90° and head is facing downwards 135° from Horizontal position (otolith debris traverse the common crus)

5. The head is kept facing to right and Patient is brought to the sitting position and head is turned forwards with chin down 20° (otolith debris enter the utricle and utricle duct) "Maintain each position for 15-20 seconds and repeated until there is no nystagmus in any position'

23

NYSTAGMUS

FEATURE OF NYSTAGMUS

1. Grading I - On looking towards the fast component

   II - On looking straight

   III - On looking towards the slow component

2. Ewald's Law I - Head and Eye movements occurs in direction of Endolymph flow & plane of the semicircular canals

   II- Lateral Semicircular canal -Ampulla pedal flow

   III- Anterior and posterior semicircular canal – Ampullo fugal flow

3. Alexander's Law - Vestibular Nystagmus increased by moving eyes in fast phase and decreased by moving eyes in slow phase

4. Null point - Position at which the Nystagmus is least marked

5. Nystagmus only when Eye fixation is removed by Frenzel glasses

MECHANISM OF LABYRINTHINE NYSTAGMUS

1. If lesion on right side vestibular nuclei (Labyrinth)

2. Decreased Tone in Right medial Rectus & Left Lateral rectus leads to slow component to right side

3. Central nervous system compensated the fast component to left side

4. Nystagmus will reduce to stage II

5. Slow component is pathological & fast component is the corrective component

CAUSES OF INDUCED NYSTAGMUS

1. Dix-Hallpike Maneuver (Positional test)

2. Fistula test

3. Tullio phenomenon

4. Caloric & Rotational test

5. Optokinetic drum & Pendulum tracking test

VARIANTS OF NYSTAGMUS

1. Erholung towards the healthy Ear within hours

    Beating towards the healthy Ear within hours

    Following attacks of Meniere's attack

2. Brunn's Nystagmus – Direction changing

    Nystagmus seen in acoustic tumor

3. See-Saw nystagmus – Optic chiasm lesions

4. Downbeat nystagmus – Arnold Chiari malformation

    Upbeat Nystagmus – Tegmentum lesions

5. Miner's Nystagmus – Occupational disease

    Peculiar to workers in coal mines in which the illumination is deficient.

24

MOTION SICKNESS

1. Kinetosis or sopite syndrome is induced when an individual is exposed to certain types of real or apparent motion stimuli

2. Clinical features are epigastric discomfort, Nausea, Pallor, Sweating, warmth body, salivation, headache, dizziness and vomiting

3. Theories are vestibular overstimulation and neural mismatch theory

    Due to visual vestibular mismatch type I & Type II with or without otolith displacement

4. Behavioral measure prevents the sickness -position at center of gravity,

    -do not do head movement,

    -closing eyes and -forward view

5. -Hyoscine 0.4 mg - 30-60 minutes before journey

    -Meclizine 25 mg - One hour before journey

    -Promethazine 25 mg - 2 Hour before journey

    -Dimenhydrinate - 4 to 8 hour before journey

    -Cinnarizine - One hour before journey

"Mal De debarquement syndrome – A persistence Vertigo by feeling of Oscillation like bobbing or swaying after landing from ship or train"

25

TRAUMA OF EAR

TRAUMATIC PERFORATION OF THE TYMPANIC MEMBRANE

1. The tendency to Tympanic membrane rupture increases with age due to air pressure, Fluids and solid objects

2. An irregular perforation occurs mostly in Anteroinferior quadrant of pars tensa and unlikely in pare flaccida

3. Caused by A blow in the ear, blast injury, barotrauma, N2o anesthesia, hyperbaric oxygen and lightning

4. Directing the jet of water on to the posterior meatal wall reduces the rupture of Tympanic membrane while ear syringing

5. Ear should not be cleaned and No ear drops advice. The perforation closes itself spontaneously within 3-6 months. If it fails, Myringoplasty can be done.

TEMPORAL BONE FRACTURE

1. Classified into longitudinal, transverse and mixed fracture

2. Longitudinal fracture (80%) -due to blows from parietal area, fracture starts in squamous part of temporal bone extends along the roof of EAC, tearing the meatal skin and Tympanic membrane and crossing the roof of the middle ear, anterior to labyrinthine through the carotid canal to end near the Foramen Spinosum or lacerum

3. Transverse (20%) -fracture due to blows from frontal or occipital areas, it begins at the jugular foramen extends across the petrous pyramid to the area of foramen spinosum and lacerum. The fracture actually traverses the Otic capsule

4. Conduction hearing loss, hemotympanum, Tympanic membrane rupture and rarely CSF with normal facial nerve in longitudinal fracture

5. SNHL, Nystagmus, Facial paralysis and CSF otorrhea seen in transverse fracture

FINDINGS OF TEMPORAL BONE

1. Perforation of the TYMPANIC MEMBRANE and meatal damage

2. Hemotympanum

3. Facial Nerve injury

4. Vestibular nerve Injury

5. Auditory nerve injury & CSF leak

LABYRINTHINE TRAUMA IN TYMPANOPLASTY

1. The removal of cholesteatoma matrix and granulation from a labyrinthine fistula (Lateral Semicircular Canal)

2. Rupture of the membranous labyrinth or labyrinthitis

3. The removal of granulations, tympanosclerosis or cholesteatoma from the oval window with fracture of stapes footplate or rupture of annular ligament

4. Excessive movement of stapes footplate or perilymph fistula

5. Contact between a toothed rotating burr and any part of an intact ossicular chain (body of incus)

26

OTOLOGICAL PROCEDURE

EAR SYRINGING

1. Simpon's syringe is used to remove earwax and foreign bodies.

2. Sterile water (normal saline 150 ml) should be at body temperature.

3. Direction of water towards posterior superior canal walls to push the wax forward or outward, to avoid direct trauma to the tympanic membrane.

4. Should not perform in case of perforated tympanic membrane and otitis externa.

6. Side effects are vasovagal shock, rupture of tympanic membrane, bleeding and vertigo.

SIEGEL'S PNEUMATIC SPECULUM

1. Magnification of 10 diopter power convex lenses used.

2. Magnified 2.5 times view of tympanic membrane and external auditory canal.

3. Mobility of the tympanic membrane.

4. Medication to apply ear drops by displacement method and to suction out the secretion from the middle ear.

5. Make out the fistula of the inner ear.

TUNING FORK TEST BASIC

1.   Rinne's test is likely to become negative at an air- bone gap of 18 dB.

2.   A lateralized Weber's test in conductive deafness may indicate a hearing loss of only 5-10 dB.

3.   Causes of lateralization

     1. Ambient sound theory.

     2. Theory of dispersion.

4.   512 Hz used because

     1. Falls under speech frequency range. (500 to 2000 Hz)

     2. Sound lasts longer for one minute.

     3. Produces less overtones (Frequencies above the fundamental frequency).

5.   Rinne test, If 256 Hz is negative - Mild 25-45 dB loss.

     If 512 Hz is negative -moderate 40-55 dB loss

     If 1024 Hz is negative- Severe hearing loss.

TUNING FORK TESTS (512 HZ)

1.   Rinne test

     -Normal is AC>BC

     -Negative is BC>AC

     Conductive hearing loss more than 25 dB

     -positive

     normal hearing or Sensorineural hearing loss

2.   Weber test -> -Conductive hearing loss more than 10-15 dB ->Lateralized to affected Ear

     - Sensorineural hearing loss -> Lateralized to normal Ear

-Centralized -> both Ears are normal

3. Absolute bone conduction test – (Modified Schwabach test) for cochlear reserve

4. Gelle test - Otosclerosis - No change in increased Air pressure in the EAC by Siegel's speculum in CHL.

5. Bing test - No change in increased Air pressure in the EAC by alternative pressure over tragus in conductive hearing loss

TESTS OF EUSTACHIAN DYSFUNCTION

1. Valsalva maneuver

2. Toynbee Maneuver

3. Frenzel Maneuver

4. Politzerization

5. Siegalisation.

CALORIC TEST (FITZGERALD - HALLPIKE BI THERMAL TEST).

1. Supine position with head elevated to an angle of 30° to bring the Lateral semicircular canal into vertical position. check the Ear for wax or Central perforation.

2. Each Ear irrigated with warm water (44°C) & cold water (30°C) in an interval of 7 Minutes for 40 Seconds duration (7°C above & below of Normal temperature)

3. "ACTH" or "COWS" -> cold produces a Nystagmus away from stimulated Ear and warm produces a nystagmus towards the stimulated Ear

4. Firstly, the affected ear is stimulated with warm water. Then the contralateral Ear is tested with warm water, then with cold water to contralateral and the test con-

cluded by cold water to the affected Ear.

5. A Normal caloric reaction in nystagmus being visible between 90 & 140 seconds after the onset of irrigation and prolongation by a further 60 seconds without visual fixation

FISTULA SIGN-HENNEBERT SIGN

1. Perilymph movement by raising air pressure produced by pressure with a finger on the tragus or pneumatic otoscope fitted with a speculum large enough to fit produces an air- tight seal.

2. On increased pressure it causes conjugate deviation of the Eye away from the examined eye due to endolymph movement towards the ampulla.

3. On maintained pressure a jerky nystagmus develops beating towards affected Ear

4. On release of pressure, the eyes return to midline as the endolymph moves away from Ampulla

5. Lateral semicircular canal fistula (Horizontal nystagmus to disease ear) Superior semicircular canal (Rotatory to normal ear) Posterior semicircular canal (Vertical nystagmus)

FALSE POSITIVE (HENNEBERT SIGN)

1. Meniere's disease

2. Hypermobility of joint plate (syphilis)

3. After stapedectomy

4. Tullio Phenomenon

5. Valsalva Induced Vertigo

FALSE NEGATIVE FISTULA TEST

1. Dead Labrinth
2. Wax
3. Cholesteatoma over fistula
4. FB
5. Anti vertigo drugs

CLINICAL TEST OF BALANCE

1. Romberg test
2. Unterberger's test
3. The gait test
4. Caloric test
5. ENG & computerized dynamic posturography

27

OTOLOGICAL SURGERY

SURGERY FOR PROTRUDING EARS

1. Converse Procedure
2. Modified converse procedure
3. Mustarde's procedure
4. Stenstrom Procedure
5. Additional procedure – Rotation of the concha and mild pressure dressing

OPERATING SCHEDULE FOR MICROTIA WITH ATRESIA AURIS

1. Unilateral microtia - > 8 yrs
2. Unilateral Atresia - Adolescence
3. Bilateral microtia - > 8 yrs
4. Bilateral Atresia- after 9-10 years
5. Reimplantation of avulsed pinna - within 24 hours microvascular anastomosis within 5 Hours of avulsion

ADVANTAGES OF LOCAL ANESTHESIA IN OTOLOGY

1. Less bleeding
2. Facial nerve function and hearing can be tested on table
3. complication of GA avoided
4. Patient can be ambulant with in a day

5. Economical

PRE OPERATIVE ADVICE FOR EAR SURGERY

1. Shampoo hair wash one day before surgery

2. Stop Aspirin, NSAID Vit E & Herbal medicine before 5 days of surgery.

3. Avoid ear bud, self -cleaning ear & ear drops.

4. Avoid cool drinks intake before 7 days of surgery

5. Bring all the reports by hand.

STEPS OF LOCAL ANESTHESIA IN OTOLOGY

1. Start T. Betaloc (Metoprolol 25 or 50 mg) bd before two days of surgery

2. Pre operative medication

   Inj. Glycopyrrolate 0.2 mg (1 amp) + Inj. Fortwin 30 mg (1 amp) +Inj. phenergan 50 mg (promethazine 2 ml), totally 5 ml given IM 45 mts before surgery.

   3. 4% Lignocaine 200 mg (5 ml) with Adrenaline 1 mg (1 amp) for peanut size cotton balls for middle ear surface anesthesia.

3. 10 ml of 2% Lignocaine with Adrenaline (1:200000) It contains 5 mcg/ml of adrenaline for Local infiltration. Only 5 ml given. Remaining 5 ml used for graft harvesting [cartilage or Fascia).

4. Start surgery after 5 minutes of Local infiltration. First infiltration around preauricular area (1 ml), second infiltration into post aural area (2 ml), finally single point Ear canal infiltration (2 ml) at 11 o'clock position (Rt ear) & 1 clock (Lt ear) just 20 mm away from Tympanic annulus than wait for 5 minutes.

POST OPERATIVE ADVICE EAR SURGERY

1. Avoid touching the operated ear or water entering the ear till 3 weeks.

2. Do not Stop any medication without informing the doctor.

3. Avoid travel and weight lifting activities

4. Avoid noisy environment

5. Avoid getting cold attacks and infection

THE BASIC PRINCIPLE OF MASTOID SURGERY

1. To eradicate active disease and thus promote the drainage and healing

2. To prevent recurrent infection

3. To prevent complications that may return

4. To restore the function

5. for ventilation

ADVANTAGES OF ENDOSCOPY IN OTOLOGY SURGERY, MAIN ADVANTAGES OF EES

1. Using the ear canal as the natural conduit to the tympanic cavity.

2. High quality resolution and magnification. Panoramic view

3. Restoring normal middle ear and mastoid ventilation routes.

4. Preserving as much as normal anatomy as possible by minimizing unnecessary

5. Dissection of bone and soft tissue, decreasing the need for drilling.

6. Avoidances of post auricular approaches and minimizing damage to neurovascular structure.

DRAWBACKS OF EES

1. Challenging one handed dissection without suction on the other hand.
2. Lack of 3 dimensional view-reliance on motion parallel to assess depth perception.
3. Lack of exposure to these techniques during surgical training.
4. Limited instrumentation.
5. Limited indication

ADVANTAGES OF MICROSCOPE IN OTOLOGY SURGERY

1. Excellent illumination.
2. Depth perception and magnification.
3. Binocular vision
4. Ability to work with 2 hands
5. Capacity to capture HD images and video

"Despite these advantages, the microscope is limited when constrained by small surgical corridors: the External auditory canal."

GOOD MASTOIDECTOMY SURGERY - (DRY MASTOID CAVITY)

1. Cavities are dry not excessively large
2. Low facial ridge
3. Adequate meatal opening
4. Closed middle ear space with adequate air

5. Retained mucosa in Mastoid air cells

BASIC PRINCIPLE OF MASTOID SURGERY

1. To Eradicate active disease (Expose, Excise & Exteriorize)
2. Promote drainage, ventilation and healing
3. To prevent recurrent infections
4. To prevent complication that might occur
5. To restore hearing function

MYRINGOPLASTY TECHNIQUE

1. Sheehy's Lateral graft
2. Glasscock's underlay Graft
3. Fisch underlay Graft
4. Sooy pedicled overlay Graft
5. Theta myringoplasty

INDICATION MYRINGOTOMY

1. Severe ear pain with bulging Tympanic membrane
2. Resistant case to antibiotics
3. Impending complication
4. Hemotympanum and 5. Diagnostic purposes.

MYRINGOTOMY

1. Anteroinferior quadrant is a site for Otitis media effusion
2. PI quadrant site for Hemotympanum.
3. Radial incision is preferred because in circular incision, the edges get inward and the Blood supply from the annulus is cut off.

4. The radial incision separates rather than cuts through fibers of the middle layer of tympanic membrane.

5. Healing is with minimal scarring in radial Incision.

INDICATION OF GROMMET TUBES

1. Chronic OME – more than 8 weeks & ASOM with complication

2. Tympanic membrane Atelectasis

3. Hemotympanum

4. ET dysfunction, Patulous ET

5. Barotrauma

PURPOSE OF GROMMET

1. Hearing Improvement.

2. Prevention of subsequent accumulation of fluid.

3. Prevention of structure damage.

4. Prevention of retraction of Tympanic membrane.

5. Alleviation of symptoms like pain, Hearing loss, tinnitus, etc.

MATERIALS FOR TYMPANIC TUBES

1. Polyethylene

2. Teflon

3. Silastic

4. Titanium

5. Silicone rubber

NAME OF TYMPANIC TUBES (DR. AG SP)

1. Donaldson, Reuter Bobbin, Reddy tubes
2. Armstrong, Air - Bel
3. Goode T, Grommet
4. Shea, Shah, Shepard
5. Paparella, Perlee, Pope

COMPLICATION OF GROMMET

1. Otorrhea
2. Myringosclerosis
3. Cholesteatoma
4. Persistent perforations
5. Trauma to ossicular chain   etc.;

GOALS OF TREATMENT IN OTITIS MEDIA

1. To make the ear safe.
2. To make the ear dry.
3. To restore the hearing.
4. To make the ear comfortable.
5. To make the ear relatively free of maintenance.

PREREQUISITES FOR MYRINGOPLASTY

1. Dry ear for 6 weeks
2. Good cochlear reserve
3. patent ET, Normal middle Ear mucosa and RW reflexes
4. ossicular chain continuity
5. No focus of infection in nose, nasopharynx & PNS.

ADVANTAGES OF MYRINGOPLASTY

1. To prevent further infection of ear
2. To improve hearing
3. To prevent tympanosclerosis
4. To enable proper fitting of hearing aid
5. To enable recruitment in certain professions like Army police ect.

ADVANTAGE OF UNDERLAY MYRINGOPLASTY

1. Lateralization and blunting are avoided.
2. Potentially less invasive.
3. Shorter healing time.
4. Less technically challenging.
5. Failures are easier to repair

THE DISADVANTAGE OF UNDERLAY MYRINGOPLASTY

1. Less exposure & middle Ear space reduced
2. More prone for adhesions with promontory.
3. Low rates of success.
4. Diseased portion of the remnant cannot be removed.
5. Less suitable for difficult cases like anterior and recurrent perforation.

ADVANTAGE OF OVERLAY MYRINGOPLASTY

1. High success rate.
2. Excellent intra operative visualization.
3. Good postoperative visualization.

4. Preservation of middle ear space.

5. No middle ear adhesions

DISADVANTAGE OF OVERLAY

1. Lateralization of the graft.

2. Squamous epidermal inclusion cyst formation.

3. healing takes a long time

4. Surgeon is inexperienced

5. Highly technically challenging.

MASTOID SURGERY INCISIONS

1. Post – Aural Incision - William Wilde

2. Modified William Wilde -incision

3. Endaural incision - Kessel – Lempert

4. Per meatal incision - Rosen

5. Cochlear implant - post aural Inverted 'U' shaped or 'L' shaped and a 'C' shaped incision.

INDICATION OF CWU [CANAL WALL UP]

1. Complication of ASOM

2. CSOM with or without cholesteatoma

3. Csf otorrhea.

4. Facial nerve trauma.

5. Neoplasm of temporal bone.

INDICATION OF CWD [CANAL WALL DOWN]

1. Large bony attic defect by cholesteatoma.

2. Extensive cholesteatoma.

3. Recurrent disease.

4. Lateral semicircular canal fistula in only hearing ear.

5. Other approaches like Glomus tumor and facial nerve decompression

INDICATION OF CORTICAL MASTOIDECTOMY

1. Acute mastoiditis.

2. Masked mastoiditis.

3. Secretory otitis media in resistant cases.

4. Chronically discharging ear with central perforation despite medical management.

5. As a preliminary step for facial nerve exposure, endo lymphatic sac decompression, cochlear implant, exposure of sigmoid sinus, petrosectomy, retro labyrinthine approaches, Trans labyrinthine approaches and combined tympanoplasty

INDICATION OF MRM

1. Unresectable disease like cholesteatoma.

2. Unreconstructable the posterior canal wall.

3. Failure of first stage cortical procedure.

4. Inadequate patient follow up.

5. Only hearing ear or dead ear

INDICATION OF RADICAL MASTOIDECTOMY

1. Peri labyrinthitis

2. Malignancy of middle ear.

3. Impending intracranial complications of CSOM

4. Cholesteatoma extending out of the middle ear.

5. Preliminary approach for glomus and facial nerve decompression.

DELAYED COMPLICATIONS OF MASTOID SURGERY

1. Posterior canal breakdown

2. Perichondritis

3. Cholesterol granuloma (leaving the blood in mastoid)

4. Mucosalization of mastoid bowl

5. Stenosis of External canal.

PER OPERATIVE COMPLICATION OF MASTOID SURGERY

1. Injury to Dura & sigmoid sinus

2. Injury to Lateral semicircular canal & short process of Incus

3. Facial nerve paralysis

4. Hearing loss

5. Dysgeusia, CSF leakage, bleeding & infection

MASTOID DRILLING TIPS

1. Always employ the microscopy, never drill the initial layer without it (unless you are an expert)

2. Drill with the widest burr possible, never drill in a burr hole. Widen the outer areas sufficiently before going deep. Burr should be TOP quality. Their sharpness should cut bone and NOT the pressure applied. If we have to apply pressure, it's time to throw away that burr (unless you are an expert)

3. A diamond burr should be reverted to when we are approaching vital structures...tegmen, sigmoid, facial nerve

4. Drill parallel to the vital structures and NEVER across it, Copious irrigation and efficient suction so that the area being drilled is constantly under our vision, is a must & reduce the thermal injury, we are unsure of an underlying structure (especially the sigmoid) we should start drilling AROUND it...if it is the sigmoid. the bluish hue would continue to unravel itself... if it's a cell the bluish hue would NOT continue and end abruptly

5. We must keep not only our eyes, but also EARS open, to appreciate the SOUND emitted by the drilling burr...the sound changes to a high pitched sound as we approach the tegmen.

TRANSTYMPANIC PERFUSION TREATMENT

1. Meniere's disease - -Gentamicin 27.6 mg/cc via 27 gauge needle - Dexamethasone 4 mg/cc for 4 weeks

2. Idiopathic Sudden Sensorineural hearing loss – Dexamethasone

3. Autoimmune inner ear disease – Dexamethasone

4. Tinnitus - Steroid 0.3 to 0.5 ml

5. The direct administration to round window membrane which diffuse into inner Ear fluids by Silverstein Micro wick self-delivery system

28

MISCELLANEOUS

NAMES AFTER MASTOID SURGERY - FIRST MASTOID SURGERY DONE BY PETIT 1736.

1. Simple mastoidectomy - Schwartze 1873

2. Modified Radical mastoidectomy - Bondy 1910 (Expose, Excise & Exteriorize)

3. Radical mastoidectomy - Kusters Stake 1889

4. Intact canal mastoidectomy - Jansen & Sheely

5. Atticotomy - Tumarkin

FIRST SURGEON IN OTOLOGY

1. Tympanoplasty - Zollner & Wullstein

2. Myringoplasty - Best Hold

3. Ossiculoplasty - Hall & Rytzner

4. Stapedectomy - Jack of Boston (Modern-shea)

5. Temporalis fascia used first by Heerman

MASTOID CAVITY OBLITERATION

1. Guildford - superior pedicle flaps

2. Palva – Post Auricular muscle

3. Meurman – Sternomastoid muscle

4. Hongkong – Temporalis fascia flap

5. Rambo – Temporalis muscle

"Elbrond flaps, Turner Temporalis double muscle flaps, Thorburn (Anteriorly based Temporalis muscle flaps), Dawlatly (posterosuperior musculofascial flaps) & Freerichs and Williams flap"

WHO COINED THE TERM IN OTOLOGY?

1. Adam Politzer   -   Otosclerosis

2. Siebenmann   -   Otospongiosis

3. Johannes Mueller   -   Cholesteatoma

4. Schuknecht   -   Keratoma, First person to use of Intratympanic injection streptomycin for Meniere's

5. Ingrassia   -   Stapes, OW, RW & Bone conduction

HISTORY IN OTOLOGY

1. First to use ear speculum   -   Guy de Chauliac

2. First Otologic head mirror   -   Hofmann 1841

3. First Audiometer   -   Hartmann 1876

4. First Cochlear implant   -   Eyrie 1957 & Djurno France

5. First ENT Specialist   -   Yearley 1850

FALLOPIUS GABRIEL NAMED

1. Cochlea & SCC

2. Tympanum

3. Chorda Tympani

4. Auditory nerve

5. Facial canal

NOBEL PRIZE IN OTOLOGY

1. Robert Barany   -   Caloric test
2. Georg Von Bekesy   -   Cochlea Mechanics
3. Emil Theodor Kocher   -   First Thyroid surgery

NORMAL VALUE IN OTOLOGY

1. Siegle's speculum magnification   - 2-2 ½ times
2. Frenzel glasses biconvex lens   - +20 Diopter
3. Thickness of silastic sheet   - 0.125 mm
4. Total volume of middle Ear   - 2 cm³
5. Normal mastoid volume   - 1 ml

OTHER VALUE

1. Impedance Compliance Normal - 0.39 ml to 1.30 ml
2. Normal middle Ear pressures   – [–] 100 mm H20 to +50 mm H2O
3. Basilar membrane length   – 13.52 mm
4. cochlear duct length   – 35 mm
5. Cochlea turns   – 2 ¾ time

Finger distance from nose (nystagmus)– 45 cm

Tuning fork kept distance from EAC – 2 cm

NONINFECTIOUS GRANULOMATOUS DISEASE OF TEMPORAL BONE

1. Wegener's Granuloma & sarcoidosis

2.   Post-Stapedectomy & Cholesterol granuloma

3.   Hand Schuller Christian disease

4.   Letterer Siwe's disease

5.   Solitary eosinophilic granuloma

(3,4,5 - Histiocytosis X Langerhans cell disorders)

INFECTIOUS GRANULOMATOUS DISEASE OF TEMPORAL BONE

1.   Tuberculosis

2.   Syphilis

3.   Leprosy

4.   Mucormycosis

5.   Cryptococcosis

29

TINNITUS

CLASSIFICATION OF TINNITUS AURIUM

1. -Subjective

   -Objective - Palatal myoclonus, Patulous eustachian tube

2. -Physiological - Brownian movement

   -Pathophysiological - Noise, Drug, Trauma

   -Pathological - Vascular, Conductive hearing loss, Sensorineural hearing loss,

   -Psychological

   -Pseudo tinnitus - Feigned, Environmental

3. Vibratory
   a) Vascular – Aneurysms, Glomus, A-V malformations
   b) Neuromuscular – Stapes muscle spasm, myoclonus — Piezoelectric, Electromagnetic, Electromechanical
   c) Miscellaneous – Patulous Eustachian tube

4. Non vibratory
   a) Presbycusis
   b) Meniere's disease
   c) Otosclerosis
   d) Diabetes mellitus, Hypothyroidism, Vitamin deficiency
   e) Bell's Palsy, Trauma Tumor

5. -Constant   - Otosclerosis

-Pulsatile- Barotrauma, Acute suppurative otitis media, Glomus

-High Pitched - drugs, Meniere's vestibular lesions

-Central Tinnitus

MEASUREMENT OF TINNITUS

Convergence
Congruence
Distance
Persistence
Divergence

1. Minimum masking level

2. Pitch match frequency

3. Tinnitus loudness Match

4. Temporal decay of masking

5. Residual inhibition

TREATMENT FOR TINNITUS (CPM HO)

1. **Counseling** (Medial, lay)

   Cochlear Iontophoresis (injection under Local Anaesthesia)

2. **Psychological**   - Cognitive, relaxation training therapy, Bio-feedback & hypnosis

3. **Medical treatment**

   a) Locozade test   - Glucose drink

   b) Anti tinnitus drug   - Clonazepam 0-5 mg

         [CSF]   - Carbamazepine 100 mg

	- Steroid 0.5-0.8 ml intratympanic
	- Flecainide 100 mg
	- Ginkgo biloba extract
4. Hearing aids	1. Improve Hearing
	2. Reduces the stress
	3. Patient Believes it is the tinnitus Which is causing the hearing difficulty
	4. Hearing aid amplified ambient noise
	5. Action of Tinnitus Masker
	a) Continues masking
	b) Inhibitory Masking
	c) DeSensitizing
5. Other	1. Electrical stimulation
	2. Ultrasonic irradiation
	3. Acupuncture
	4. Avoid of food, drink and drug
	5. Dietary Supplements
	NaF, Zinc Sulphate, Multivitamins

30

AUDIOLOGY AND HEARING AIDS

HEARING AID TYPES

1. Evolution
   1. Air conduction Mechanical
   2. Bone conduction Mechanical
   3. Electrical hearing aids
   4. Electric hearing aid
   5. Digital hearing aid

2. Mode of Placement
   1. Body worn – till 5 years
   2. In the ear, In the canal & Completely in the canal
   3. Behind the ear
   4. Implantable
      a) Middle ear implant
      b) Temporal bone stimulator
      c) Otic capsule stimulator
   5. Eye spectate aids

3. Mode of operation
   1. Single band
   2. Multi band
   3. Transpositional
   4. FM

4.	Mode of presentation	1. Air conduction
		2. Bone conduction
		3. Monaural
		4. Binaural
5.	Mode of gain	1. Low gain Hearing aid
		2. Moderate gain Hearing aid
		3. High Gain hearing aid

"CROS (Contralateral routing of signals)- BI CROS & UNI CROS

FROS (Frontal Rooting of Signals)"

INDICATION OF HEARING AID IN CONDUCTIVE HEARING LOSS

1. Bilateral otitis media, Patient refusing surgery or unfit for surgery
2. Children with bilateral conductive hearing loss until the age for surgery
3. Otosclerosis
4. Meniere's Disease
5. Tinnitus Maskers

CAUSES OF SQUEAL (LOUD HIGH NOISES FROM HEARING AID)

1. ILL Fitting ear Moulds
2. Too much amplification
3. Fluid in the middle ear
4. Wax in ear canal
5. maximum power output

THE PERCENTAGE OF HEARING IMPAIRMENT

1. If the BC level is normal (<20dBL), But

   The A-B gab is > 20 dB HL, it is Conductive hearing loss

2. If BC level is > 20 dB HL, But

   The A-B gab is < 20 dB HL, is Sensorineural hearing loss

3. If BC level is > 20 dB HL, but

   The A-B gab is > 20 dB HL is mixed hearing loss

4. Unilateral deafness

   a+b+c+d /4-25X1.5%

   a = (500 KHZ) b = (100 KH$_z$) c = (2000 KHZ) d = (3000 KHZ)

5. Bilateral deafness

   (5X+Y) ÷ 6 X (better ear %) Y (worse ear %)

VARIOUS SHAPE OF PURE TONE AUDIOGRAM

1. Right sloping Audiogram - Serous Otitis Media

   (High frequency CHL)

2. Left sloping Audiogram - Otosclerosis

   (Low frequency CHL)

3. Flat Audiogram - Strial Presbycusis, salicylate poisoning

   (Mid frequency SNHL)

4. Descending Audiogram- Ototoxic drugs, Noise induced

   (High Frequency SNHL)

5. Ascending Audiogram - Endolymphatic Hydrops

   (Low frequency SNHL)

NAMED AUDIOGRAM

1.	Trough shaped Audiogram	- Congenital SNHL
2.	'V' shaped Audiogram	- Hereditary Hearing loss
3.	Carhart's Notch (2 KH)	- Otosclerosis
4.	Acoustic Notch (4 KH)	- Noise Induced SNHL
5.	Cookie bite Audiogram	- Cochlear Otosclerosis SNHL

TONE DECAY TEST

1. The tone is heard for one full minute after raising 30 dB above the normal threshold

2. Procedure
   a) Carhart's method
   b) Green's method
   c) Olsen & Noffisinges method
   d) Rosenberg's method
   e) Supra threshold Jerges Adaptation method

3. Positive in   - Retro cochlear Pathology

4. Mechanism is like the Wedensky's Peripheral nerve inhibition

5. If tone decay

- 0 dB to 5 dB	- Normal, CHL
- Mild 10-15 dB	- Cochlear
- Moderate 20-25 dB	- Moderate
-Severe 30 dB	- Retro cochlear

USES OF AUDIOGRAM

1. To know the severity of deafness
2. To know the type of deafness
3. Gives a clue to the disease
4. Documentary
5. Variety of frequency can be tested

RECRUITMENT TEST – FOWLER 1937

1. An abnormally steep growth of Loudness with increasing intensity in cochlear pathology.
2. Presence of recruitment in SNHL

    -> Cochlear Pathology -Absence of recruitment in SNHL

    ->Retro cochlear pathology

3. **(ABLB)**Alternate Binaural Loudness Balance – Direct test in Alternate Binaural Loudness Balance, Send Two tones of the same frequency to both ears

    Absent Recruitment - SNHL with normal Cochlear

    Complete Recruitment - Cochlear Pathology

    Partial Recruitment - No Diagnostic value

    Decruitment - Subtractive Hearing loss

    ABLB plotting graph from the abscissa for poorer ear & Plotting Graph from the ladder graph for better ear

4. **SISI** – Indirect test is short increment Sensitivity index test Examines the power of the subject to detect small changes in intensity of a sound

    (example: 1 dB increment in 20 dB the threshold in various frequency)

    Positive SIS Score 70-100%   - cochlear pathology

Negative SISI score 0-20%   - retro cochlear pathology

5. Other test for recruitment

- Metz Recruitment test

- Loudness discomfort level

USES OF IMPEDANCE TESTS

1. Objective differentiation between CHL & SNHL

2. Differential diagnosis in cases of CHL

3. Measurement of middle ear pressure and Evaluation of Eustachian Tube function

4. Differential diagnosis of a SNHL whether a lesion is cochlear or retro cochlear

5. Identification of site of lesion in facial paralysis and certain brainstem Pathologies

PRINCIPLE OF TYMPANOMETRY

1. Impedance of the medium = stiffness + mass + friction. Air has low impedance cochlear fluid has a high impedance. Impedance matching measured by electroacoustic bridge which contains

    a) probe tone (p220 or 226 HZ) delivered sound

    b] Microphone amplifies measured the reflected sound

    c] Air-Pump Manometer pressure (– 600 mm of water to + 300 mm of water)

2. Admittance is reciprocal of impedance (unit is mho)

3. Compliance is reciprocal of stiffness (unit is cc or ml)

4. Acoustic compliance is an expression of the movement of middle ear system

5. The result of tympanometry when displayed graphically with impedance of stiffness of middle ear as the ordinate (Y-Axis) and air pressure as the abscissa (x-Axis) is called "Tympanogram".

DECREASED COMPLIANCE

Normal = 0.35 to 1.40 ml

1. Otosclerosis
2. Ossicular fixation like Fixed malleus syndrome
3. Serous Otitis Media or Adhesive otitis media
4. Tympanosclerosis or thickening of TM
5. Tumors in the middle ear-glomus

INCREASED COMPLIANCE

1. Ossicular discontinuity
2. Scarring Tm
3. Large TM
4. Post – stapedectomy ear
5. Healed TM

ABSENCE OF ANY PRESSURE PEAK

Normal pressure (- 50 mm of water to +50 mm of water)

1. Adhesive otitis media
2. Perforation of TM
3. Patent Grommet
4. Wax
5. Artifact by probe tip

NORMAL MIDDLE EAR PRESSURE

1. Otosclerosis
2. Ossicular discontinuity
3. Fixed malleus
4. Scarring TM
5. Healed TM

TYPE AND SHAPE OF TYMPANOGRAM

(Jerger's type)

1. Type A   - Normal tympanogram
2. Type AS   - Small or short peak – Otosclerosis
   Type Ad   - Deep peak – Ossicular discontinuity
3. Type B - Secretory otitis media, flat tympanogram
4. Type C - Blocked Eustachian tube, Scarring TM
5. Type E - Broad deep Notching by 660 H_z - Ossicular discontinuity

ACOUSTIC STAPEDIAL REFLEX

(Sound to Ear above 90 dB)

1. Receptor   - Organ of Corti
2. Afferent   - VII CN to cochlear Nucleus
3. Centre   - Superior olivary complex in brainstem
4. Efferent   - Both sides of VII C.N. Motor nucleus
5. Response   - Stimulation of Both Stapedius muscle

   Leads contraction of muscle which pulls the stapes slightly inward & outward

ADVANTAGE OF STAPEDIAL REFLEX DETECTION

1. Simple to perform, need little time, non-invasive, objective response and carried on New-born Babies also

2. Elimination of middle Ear pathology

3. Differentiation of cochlear & retro cochlear Pathology

4. Identifying the level of lesion of VII CN Paralysis

5. Defection of non-organic hearing loss

INTERPRETATION OF ACOUSTIC REFLEX

1. Unilateral CHL – The contralateral as well as ipsilateral reflexes will be absent in deaf ear but in the normal ear the ipsilateral reflex will be present and the contralateral reflex will be absent

2. Bilateral CHL – Absent with ipsilateral & contra bilaterally

3. Unilateral SNHL – Reflex will be present in the deaf ear only on contralateral stimulation.

4. Bilateral SNHL – Bilaterally present on both ipsilateral & contralateral stimulation in cochlear lesion due to loudness recruitment

    - Reflexes absent in retro cochlear lesion

5. Central lesions – Example; brainstem multiple sclerosis Reflexes are present bilaterally on ipsilateral stimulation only but absent bilaterally on contralateral stimulation

USES OF BERA (JEWETT 1970)

1. Detection deafness in infants, mentally retarded, malingering, deeply sedated & Anesthetized patients

2. Assessment of the nature of deafness like CHL, SNHL

3. Identification of the site of lesion in retro cochlear pathology [cochlear nerve, cochlear nucleus, superior olivary, lateral lemniscus and inferior colliculus]

4. Central Auditory disorders

5. Brain death, assessing prognosis in Coma patient

PRINCIPLE OF BERA

1. Brainstem Evoked Response Audiometry is graphic recording by click like sound stimulus above 60 dB of the average pure tone hearing level

2. First 10 milliseconds recording gives 5 to 7 waves of early latency response

3. The reference electrode is placed on the testing ear mastoid, and a ground electrode is placed over the forehead.

4. Latency, amplitude, wave morphology & (LAW) are studied, Latency -intensity function of wave V also studied.

5. Middle latency response (80 MS)

   Late Latency Response (500 MS)

   Also recorded some time.

BERA WAVES

5 Prominent peaks (I to V)

2 Small peaks (A and B)

WAVE Site (CNSLI)

1. I- Distal End of cochlear nerve. Latency - 1.65 s

   If wave I is present but other waves absent -> cochlea is normal

   So, Retro cochlear pathology

If wave I is delayed but others are normal -> CHL or Cochlear pathology

2. II- Cochlear nucleus   -2 ms
3. III- Superior olivary complex -3.70 ms
4. VI- Lateral lemniscus   -4.84 ms
5. V- Inferior colliculus   -5.56 ms there is sharp negative deflection of wave

PARAMETERS OF BERA

1. Inter Latency between wave I & V is 4 ms
2. Inter aural latency of two ear is 0.2 ms
3. Time interval between (V) I & III is increased in acoustic neuroma (normal 2 ms)
4. Increase Latency and decreased Amplitude in multiple sclerosis
5. Inter peak latency between III to V is 2 ms

QUANTITY THE DEAFNESS

1. 25 dB   - Normal
2. 26 to 40 dB   - Mild deafness
3. 41 to 55 dB   - Moderate deafness
4. 56 to 70 dB   - Moderately severe deafness
5. 71 to 90 dB   - Very severe deafness

    above 90 dB   - profound deafness

SPEECH AUDIOMETRY

1. The identification of neural types of hearing loss in both the reception (SRT)as well as the discrimination (SDS) of speech.

2. SRT (Speech Reception Threshold) – 6 spondee words (Example; baseball, horseshoe) present above 25 dB of SRT

   If 50% of words correctly identified is normal

   SRT is poorer in neural lesions

3. SDS (Speech discrimination score) – Phonetically balanced word monosyllabic

   Words like as, can, age present above 35 dB of SRT

   The % of the total number of words identified

   gives SD score

   SDS

0-30%	-	Retro cochlear lesion
30-85%	-	Cochlear lesion
>85%	-	Normal (90-100%)

4. Rollover ration= Less than 0.4 is cochlear lesion

   = more than 0.4 is neural lesion

5. Criteria for speech Audiometry

   a. Using only standardized word – lists (Spondee & PB)

   b. Mother tongue

   c. Two room set up

   d. Live voice

   e. Sound-free test environment

BEKESY AUDIOMETRY

Self-Recording Audiometry

1. Type   I   Overlap of pulsed and continuous recording – Normal or CHL

2. Type II   Normal up to 1 KHz, above which the continuous trace falls away from the pulse trace – cochlear

3. Type III   Continuous trace falls rapidly away – neural lesions

4. Type IV   Continuous trace runs below the pulsed trace from above 500 Hz

5. Type V   Continuous trace above the pulse trace non-organic hearing loss

AUDIOMETRY IN CHILDREN

1. Free field audiometry

2. Behavioral observation Audiometer

3. Visual reinforcement Audiometry

4. Play Audiometry

5. Tangible reinforcement operant conditioning Audiometry

AUDIOMETRY TEST FOR FEIGNING OR MALINGERING DEAFNESS

1. Erhad's lord voice test   - Occlusion of meatus

2. Lombard's voice reflex test   - Loud reading

3. Hummel's double conversation test - Two speaker

4. Teuber's voice test   - Tube

5. Callahan's voice test & Doerfler – stewart test

ELECTROCOCHLEOGRAPHY

1. The electrical activity generated by the cochlea and in the auditory nerve can be measured by a system called

electrocochleography by placing an active electrode on promontory or Round Window under Anesthesia or non-invasively by placing over Tympanic membrane.

2. The Parametric are

   a. Cochlear microphonic arising in vicinity hair cell (CM)

   b. Summating potential arising in the inner hair cell (SP)

   c. Auditory nerve compound action potential (AP) sum of the discharge of the whole of the cochlear nerve

3. -Normal SP/AP ratio is 0.3 to 0.5 (<0.4) -normal SP amplitude and AP amplitude is 20%

   - E COG recording within first 3 milliseconds after clicks

4. The mechanism of enlarged SP appears to be displacement of basilar membrane towards scala tympani which is induced by hydrops

5. Uses of EcochG

   a. Diagnosis Of Meniere's disease

   b. Ascertaining the hearing threshold

   c. Monitoring the integrity of the cochlea & cochlear nerve during oto neurological surgery

   d. Helping interpretation of BERA is Case where the wave I of BERA is not identifiable and e. For differential Diagnosis of various type of SNHL

OTOACOUSTIC EMISSIONS - DAVID KEMP 1978

1. The sound emitted by the normal cochlea which can be picked-up recorded and measured by placing a microphone – receiver in the deep external meatus

2. Its objective screening of hearing in neonates since it is very sensitive, non-invasive requires 5 minutes only

3. Types of OAE

   a. Spontaneous OAE in absence of any stimulus seen in 50% of normal cochlear

   b. Evoked OAE are elicited by click sound 80 dB at intervals of 20 ms – 90 to 100% normal cochlea

      i. Transient OAE   - Normal to mild HL

      ii. Distortion OAE   - Elicited by two stimulus tones separated in frequency (2F1-F2) it is free from Artifacts and is present till 60 dB in Sensorineural loss

4. Uses of OAE

   a. To differentiate cochlear and cochlear pathology

   b. Early changes of ototoxicity can be detected

   c. To rule out malingering

   d. Intra operative monitoring

   e. Monitor Meniere's disease

5. Disadvantages- may miss mild hearing loss, can't quantify hearing loss & Not useful in central Auditory pathology

TESTS RESULTS FOR COCHLEAR LESIONS

1. PTA -Low frequency SNHL & rising Audiogram pattern

2. Recruitment test

   Acoustic reflex test   Present

   Diplacusis

   SISI-High Score

3. Reflex decay

Tone decay   Absent

4. Speech discrimination

Dynamic range

ART-PTT   Decreased

Upper comfortable Level

5. ABLB

LI Function curve   Converging

TESTS RESULTS FOR RETRO COCHLEAR PATHOLOGY

1. PTA   - High frequency SNHL & Convergent Audiogram pattern

2. Recruitment test

Acoustic reflex test   Absent

Diplacusis

SISI-Poor Score

3. Speech discrimination

Dynamic range

ART-PTT   Increased

Upper comfortable Level

4. Reflex decay

Tone decay   Present

5. ABLB

LI Function curve   Diverging

NEURAL RESPONSE TELEMETRY – CARTER 1995 BASED ON BROWN 1990

1. In situ Intracochlear recordings of the electrically evoked compound action potential from the Auditory nerves using scala tympani electrodes

2. Used in

   a. Information about the degree of neural survival in the stimulated cochlea

   b. If determining optimal speech coding parameters for cochlear implant users on individual basis

   c. Recording done at intra operative or postoperative

3. It needs nucleus 24 system & NRT software to record the waves by stimulation of (IPS) Interface cord to process or control interface to sprint to Radiofrequency coils which received by Implant leads to AP recorded same was recorded by NRT software and stored in PC

4. NRT wave forms a) Negative wave (N_1) b) Single positive (P_1) c) double positive peak (P_2) N_1P_1 category are Ia, Ib, Ic, P2 category is II

5. All 22 stimulation recording done from electrode I is made basal site and electrode 22 is most apical one is the array

ELECTRONYSTAGMOGRAPHY

1. It is useful qualitative and quantitative objective information about Nystagmus. The subject's Eyes closed is a major advantage. Frenzel's glasses

2. It allows measurement various nystagmus parameter like slow phase velocity, amplitude, frequency, duration, fast phase velocity, total numbers of beats & latency

3. ENG cannot record nystagmus in blindness where the Corneo retinal potential is absent and purely rotational nystagmus

4. ENG tracing is triangular with one basal angle greater than the other, it must have a slow phase & a fast phase. Its amplitude should be more than 20 mv

5. A movement of the eyes to the right is recorded as an upward deflection of the writing needle and a movement to the left as a downward deflection

AIM OF ENG

1. Any abnormality in the vestibular system

2. Is this peripheral or central vestibular system

3. If it is peripheral, which side is involved

4. If it in central site of involved like brainstem, cerebellum & cerebral

5. Is the lesion static, progressive or recovering?

VEMP

1. Vestibular evoked myogenic potentials are short latency vestibular dependent reflexes that are recorded from the SCM (sternocleidomastoid) in the anterior neck (Cervical or cVEMP) and the inferior oblique extra ocular muscle [ocular Vemps or oVEMP). They are evoked but short bursts of sound delivered through headphones or vibration applied to the skull. VEMPs are used clinically as measures of otolith function

2. cVemp (Colebatch 1994) is a biphasic surface potential, with peaks at 13 & 23ms recorded from electrodes arranged in a belly-tendon montage

over sternocleidomastoid as air – conducted sound preferentially activates the saccule (ipsilateral reflex)

3. oVEMP (Rosengren 2005) originates in inferior oblique muscle & is produced by a brief excitation of the muscle. The response peaks at 10 & 15ms beginning with a negativity. It used clinically to assess the function of the utricle (Contralateral reflex)

4. VEMPS Results

   a. Acute vestibular syndrome- Absent or reduced.

   b. Ac & BC oVEMP in presence of preserved AC, cVEMP

   c. BPPV – Elevated rates of VBMP abnormity

   d. Vestibular Migraine – Normal Response.

   e. Menere's –c Vemp reduced in affected ear while positive oVemp are preserved bilateral

   f. Superior canal dehiscence – Large oVemp& cVemp with high Amplitude

   g. Unilateral vestibular loss(schwannoma)-Reduced

VHIT

1. The video head impulse test is quantitative assessment of the positive Vestibulo-ocular reflex, in vHIT eye movements are recorded and analyzed by high speed cameras & head movements are measured by motion sensors embedded in the vHIT goggles

2. In normal impulses at less than 150 degrees/sec the head and VOR gain is approximately equal to one

3. Used   a) Identify isolated abnormalities in vertical canal

   b) Serial testing in Gentamicin in Meniere's

c) In patients with bilateral caloric weakness

d) Differentiate peripheral vestibular disorders from stroke in acute persistence vertigo.

4. VHIT Vs caloric test.

5. To interpret to catch-up the saccade consider frequency, Direction, Latency & Velocity